THE BEST VAGINA:

The secret to a Joyful vagina and Guide
to women's health; solution to dryness
and infection free vagina.

By

Sadie B. Allen.

0

Copyright

About the Author

Hot advocate for women's health and autonomy, Sadie B. Allen, wrote "The Best Vagina." Bringing a fresh and informative perspective to the conversation around women's specific health, Allen has a history in both sexual virility and education. She uses a combination of wisdom, humor, and evidence-based guidance in her work to guide readers toward a more fulfilling and positive relationship. With "The Stylish Vagina," Allen wants to dispel myths, educate readers, and encourage a positive relationship with one's body. Accompany her on her transformative journey towards self-discovery and optimal health and wellness.

Table of Content

Introduction: The Vagina

An essential component of your internal and exterior reproductive anatomy is the vagina. This text has significant implications for menstruation, sex, pregnancy, and labor. Maintaining a healthy and infection-free vagina can be achieved with routine pelvic exams, Pap screenings, and safer sexual behaviors.

Who's got a vagina?

Individuals classified as female at birth (AFAB) possess vaginas. People who identify as AFAB and are cisgender women, as well as some transgender men and nonbinary people, are considered AFAB. Some intersex people also have cervixes.

Some nonbinary people who identify as transgender and who are not AFAB decide to undergo vaginoplasty, a gender-affirming procedure. Through a vaginoplasty, a person's genitalia are transformed into a vagina.

Operation

How does the vagina function?

In addition to facilitating sexual pleasure, your vagina also plays a part in pregnancy and childbirth by directing your menstrual blood outside of your body.

Sexual pleasure: When a penis, a finger, or a sex toy penetrates your vagina, nerve endings within the walls of your vagina allow you to feel pleasure. When you're aroused, your vagina enlarges and lubricates itself to keep the friction from being painful rather than enjoyable.

Menstruation: Unless you become pregnant, you lose the endometrium, or lining of your uterus, once a month during your menstrual cycle. Menstrual blood leaves your body through your vagina, carrying the lining. Tampons and menstrual cups are useful tools for controlling vaginal blood flow.

Pregnancy: If your partner ejaculates during penis-in-vagina sex (intercourse), sperm may be released into your vaginal canal. To fertilize an egg, sperm must swim from your vagina through your uterus and fallopian tubes.

Childbirth: When discussing the vagina's function during childbirth, people occasionally refer to it as a "birth canal." To be born, your baby must pass through your vagina after leaving your uterus. The final stop on your baby's journey from your body to the outside world is your vaginal opening.

Fascinating details about your vagina

Because a vagina cleans itself without assistance, it is sometimes compared to a self-cleaning oven. Numerous bacteria and fungi inhabit your vagina, maintaining its health. Vaginal flora, also known as your microbiome, is the delicate ecosystem in which these microscopic organisms live. Your vagina is free of infections when the proper balance of these organisms—particularly a large number of Lactobacilli, the "good" bacteria—are present. An overabundance of fungi or an unbalanced bacterial population can cause an infection.

Anatomy

Where is the vagina in your body?

"Vaginas" and "vulvas" are often confused, but they are not the same thing. Your vagina is an organ that resembles a canal that is inside of you and opens externally. It's a strong passage that connects your vulva, or external reproductive organs, to your uterus, which is located inside your body.

Within Your Body

Your cervix, a tissue structure that resembles a neck and joins your vagina to your uterus, is where your vagina extends from. Your vagina terminates at your vaginal opening, which is a hole outside of your body. The rectum, which houses your feces, and the bladder, which holds your urine, or pee, is separated by the vagina.

Situated on the front wall, a few inches inside your vagina, is where your G-spot is. During sex, many people find it enjoyable to stimulate this area with their finger or penis.

Beyond your body

Your vulva contains a hole known as your vaginal opening, where your vagina ends. The folds of skin on either side of your vaginal opening are called vulva. The labia majora are the outer folds. Your labia minora, or inner lips, are the inner folds. Where your inner lips converge towards the top of your vulva is where your clitoris, or clit, is situated. Where your inner lips meet towards the base of your vulva is where your vaginal opening is found. Your vaginal opening may occasionally be fully or partially covered by your inner lips. To feel your vaginal opening, you might need to use your fingers to part your inner lips.

One of the three vital openings in your vulva region that connects the internal and external functions of your body is your vaginal opening. On top is your urethral opening. It is your vaginal opening in the center. Your anus is located at the base.

Urethral opening: The tiny opening that permits urination beneath your clitoris. At this opening, the urethra, the tube that carries urine from your bladder, empties into the outside world.

Vaginal opening: This is the opening through which your baby leaves your body during childbirth and through which menstrual blood flows. It's also the opening through which a menstruation cup, tampon, penis, finger, or sex toy can be inserted. Your vaginal opening is often covered, or partially covered, by a thin membrane known as a hymen. This membrane can get strained when you exercise, have sex, or even put a tampon in. It might hurt to stretch like this or it might not.

Anus: This opening is where the organ that transports waste from your colon (rectum) exits your body.

What is a vagina's average depth?

When not aroused, the average vagina is slightly deeper than 3.5 inches. However, a number of factors, such as your age, weight, and menopause status, affect how big your vagina is. The total length of your vagina may also get shorter after pelvic cavity surgeries.

Your vagina is a flexible organ that has a maximum depth that it can reach. The organ known as the cervix, which joins your vagina to your uterus, tilts upward when you become aroused, lengthening your vaginal canal in the process. You can stretch your vagina to accommodate a finger, penis, or sex toy. Even so, if something is inserted and comes into contact with your cervix, the experience may become uncomfortable. Talk to your partners about what makes you feel good.

What composes the vagina?

The vagina is made up of various tissue and cell types that secrete fluids to maintain the moisture, elasticity, and health of the vaginal walls. The hormone estrogen has a particularly strong effect on the cells in your vagina. During your reproductive years, your body produces more estrogen than it does during menopause. Following menopause, your vaginal walls may thin and become dry due to a decrease in estrogen. When vagina becomes dry after menopause, over-the-counter lubricants and estrogen replacement therapy can help.

Disorders and Conditions

Which common ailments and conditions affect your vagina?

Your vagina can be affected by a number of conditions, but vaginitis—a group of illnesses that result in vaginal inflammation and/or infection—is the most typical issue. The most prevalent ailments covered by this broader category are:

Bacterial vaginosis: An infection of the vaginal flora brought on by an overabundance of bacteria, particularly Gardnerella vaginalis.

Vaginal yeast infections: A vaginal infection caused by an overgrowth of candida yeast in the vagina.

Trichomonas vaginalis is the parasite that causes trichomoniasis, a sexually transmitted infection (STI).

Additional prerequisites consist of:

A fluid-filled sac known as a bartholin cyst can develop on the gland called the Bartholin, which is situated on either side of the vaginal opening.

Chlamydia: A bacteria known as Chlamydia trachomatis is the source of this sexually transmitted infection (STI).

Herpes simplex virus (HSV) is the source of genital herpes, a STI.

A STI known as gonorrhea is brought on by the bacteria Neisseria gonorrhoeae.

Human papillomavirus infection: A sexually transmitted infection.

A STI known as syphilis is brought on by the bacteria Treponema pallidum.

Vaginal atrophy: A condition that develops after menopause in which a decrease in estrogen causes your vaginal walls to thin and dry out.

Vaginal cancer: An uncommon kind of cancer that primarily affects those who have had HPV infections.

Vulvar cancer: An uncommon form of cancer brought on by lichen sclerosus or HPV infection.

A condition known as vaginal prolapse occurs when the pelvic floor muscles weaken and cause the vagina to slide out of position.

What are typical symptoms or indicators of vaginal disorders?

The symptoms you experience will vary based on the nature of your particular condition. Particularly, changes in your vaginal discharge typically indicate the presence of an infection.

Heavy menstrual flow or irregular vaginal bleeding.

Vaginal discharge that can appear green, gray, off-white, or clear.

The consistency of vaginal discharge resembles cottage cheese.

Fishy-smelling vaginal discharge.

Vulva or vaginal itching, burning, or soreness.

Burning feeling after urinating.

Dysentery during sexual activity.

Which tests are commonly used to assess the health of the vagina?

Pelvic exam: Your doctor examines your vulva and vagina to look for anomalies or illness-related symptoms.

Pap smear: A test used to look for cervical cancer indicators. Rarely, aberrant Pap tests could point to vaginal cancer symptoms. Rarely, aberrant Pap tests could point to vaginal cancer symptoms.

Colposcopy: A procedure in which the tissue in your vagina is magnified using a special lighted microscope. Any questionable areas on your vagina can be sampled by your healthcare provider, who can then test the tissue in a lab.

Test that determines your PH levels, or how acidic your vaginal fluids are: the vaginal pH test. Your physician can diagnose an infection with the aid of your PH levels.

STI tests: To look for the microorganisms that cause STIs, your doctor may perform a urine (urinalysis) or vaginal fluid test.

Pelvic imaging: Your doctor may request an imaging test in order to vagina for tumors or structural issues such as prolapse. The most popular test performed is an ultrasound, but your doctor may also order computed tomography (CT) and magnetic resonance imaging (MRI).

Biopsy: To check for cancer cells, your healthcare provider might remove a sample of tissue.

Which common treatments are administered for your vagina?

The majority of vaginitis causes can be treated with antifungal drugs or antibiotic gels, creams, and pills. Hormone therapy frequently improves vaginal abnormalities like vaginal atrophy that are caused by estrogen reductions.

Surgery or other treatments like radiation and chemotherapy may be necessary for vaginal cancer. The degree of cancer determines the course of treatment.

Take Care

Easy lifestyle choices to maintain the health of your vagina

Achieve routine Pap smears and pelvic exams. Not every vaginal condition has symptoms that are obvious. Frequent screenings enable your healthcare provider to identify problems early and take appropriate action.

Refrain from douching. The delicate balance of bacteria in your vaginal flora that prevents infections can be upset by douching.

Take off any sweaty or damp clothes. Your chance of developing a bacterial or fungal infection can be decreased by wearing dry clothes.

Exercise your pelvic floor (Kegel exercises). Regular pelvic floor exercise can help prevent diseases like vaginal prolapse. Your ability to control and squeeze your vaginal walls is enhanced by having strong pelvic floor muscles, which also heightens the pleasure of arousal and orgasm.

Have safer sexual relations. When engaging in oral, anal, or intercourse, use condoms or dental dams. Limit the number of sex partners you have and refrain from sharing sex toys. You can lower your risk of infection with safer sex.

A message from Cleveland Clinic

As a component of your internal and external reproductive organs, your vagina is essential. The vagina facilitates sexual pleasure, pregnancy, and childbirth. To lower your risk of infection, take better care of your vagina by having safer sexual relations. Steer clear of douching, as this may interfere with your vagina's ability to clean itself. To make sure your vagina stays healthy, schedule routine pelvic exams with your healthcare provider.

Chapter 1: Vagina Health

It is surprisingly simple to maintain good vulva and vaginal health. Knowing what works for you and your body is the first step. If something seems off, consult your OB-GYN provider.

Contrary to what you may have read, adequate vulva and vaginal care does not require any specific products. Actually, your vagina was designed to clean itself; your main responsibility is to keep an eye on and maintain a clean, healthy environment around you.

Let's go over the fundamentals before going over some advice for good hygiene habits that will promote the healthiest vulva and vagina.

Vulva versus vagina

Surprisingly, a lot of women mix up vulva and vagina. Let's recap the two different areas of female genitalia.

What is meant by the vulva?

Your vulva encloses and shields your urethra, the opening to your urinary system, as well as your external genitalia, which include your labia, pubic mound, clitoris, and opening to the vagina.

What is meant by the vagina?
The vulva is connected to the cervix and, eventually, to the uterus through the vagina. The canal makes monthly menstruation and childbirth possible.

Now that we are using the proper language, let's go over some advice for preserving the best possible vulva and vaginal health.

1. **Maintaining Order**: It is easy to clean your vulvovaginal area:

1. **Wash every day in warm water**; you can use a mild soap, such as Pears, Basis, Neutrogena, or Dove-Hypoallergenic, but it's not necessary. Grab a pair of fingers rather than a washcloth.

2. **Avoid washing your vagina inside out**. If you do, it might throw off its delicate pH balance and cause infection and irritability. Usually, vaginal discharge serves as self-cleansing.

3. **Steer clear of douching, scented soaps**, and special scrubs—even those that claim to be made for vaginal care. These may also cause an infection and upset your body's natural pH balance. First of all, if you're worried about vaginal odors, keep in mind that the vagina is not and was never meant to be a flower. But you should call your Moreland OB-GYN physician if you smell something

different than your typical "Eau de you" and feel burning, itching, or other discomforts.

4. **Wipe the front and then the back after using the restroom**. Reversing the process could result in an infection of the urinary tract by transferring bacteria to the urethra.

2. Clean, Pleasureful Intercourse

Your vulva is a significant source of gratification, so it's critical to keep it free from dangerous substances and germs.

Prior to

Inspect the components of any lubricants you intend to apply. Some might include unwholesome components that upset your pH equilibrium. Steer clear of lubricants containing:

Glycerin

- Petroleum-based goods
- Paraben-containing
- Aromas
- Tastes
- Artificial oils
- Colors

1. A few doctor-approved lubricant varieties are available at Moreland OB-GYN. In our office, we quietly sell these. Together with your provider, you can go over the options to determine which one best suit your needs.

2. Verify the contents of condoms as well. Many brands contain spermicides, which can destroy the beneficial bacteria in your vagina, throw off the pH balance, irritate your skin, and cause infection.

While

Use a fresh condom each time you switch between vaginal and anal sex, or vice versa. Similar to how your vagina has bacteria that can irritate your anus, your anus can harbor strains of bacteria that can infect or irritate your vagina.

Following

Urinate after sex to remove any bacteria that may have entered the urethra and prevent getting a urinary tract infection.

After giving the vulva a warm water shower or cleaning, make sure the area is fully dry.

3. Put on Success-Oriented Clothing

Wear clothes that will allow the area around your vulvovaginal to breathe easily and stay dry. A yeast infection may result from the growth of bacteria, which is encouraged by moisture.

Put on cotton underwear instead of polyester or silk. Cotton is less likely to retain moisture and hinders the growth of bacteria that cause odors. If you'd prefer a more open fit around your legs, check out women's boyshorts.

Steer clear of tight clothing, especially thongs, as they can gather excrement that can enter the vagina and lead to infections and bad smells.

After working out, change into clean clothes and underwear.

Steer clear of swimming in a wet suit all day.

Swap your underwear twice a day if you have a lot of vaginal discharge.

Eliminate perspiration around the vulva during the night by not wearing any underwear at all.

4. Should I Shave My Pubic Hair?

The vulva is shielded from bacteria and viruses by its pubic hair. It cushions and shields the delicate skin it covers from rubbing during intercourse. Pubic hair does not present a health risk if it is cleaned on a regular basis.

Some women would rather get rid of their pubic hair entirely through electrolysis, waxing, or shaving because they believe it causes more moisture and odor. Some believe that trimming it with scissors and keeping it well-groomed helps to lessen those issues. Some people would rather keep it natural. You really do have a choice.

Razor burn, redness, itching when hair grows back, and infections from ingrown hairs can all result from shaving. Unwanted bacteria can also enter cuts and nicks. Hair removal cream can be particularly harsh on the vulva's delicate skin and burns off hair, so avoid using it.

5. Typical Vaginal Cleaning

Here are some more pointers for maintaining healthy vulvovaginal health: Untitled artwork

Avoid using tampons, pads, and liners that have scents.

When you're on your period, change your tampon four to five times a day. This holds true for pads and liners as well.

Make sure to wash or wipe the area frequently while you're menstruating.

Eating probiotics, such as yogurt, can help reduce vaginal odor and prevent yeast infections by preserving the right pH balance in your vagina. Don't put yogurt in your private parts! Actually, the sugars in it may encourage the growth of yeast.)

Keeping yourself properly hydrated helps manage the growth of bacteria and stress-related sweating.

Attend any follow-up appointments if you have any concerns, as well as your yearly wellness visit with your Moreland OB-GYN doctor.

6. Urinating after sexual activity can reduce the risk of UTIs after having sex. It also lets you arrange for some personal cleanup time.

7. Get into bed wearing your birthday suit.

It's true that your vagina can benefit from sleeping bare. Regardless of what you wear during the day, wearing nothing underwear overnight can help with vaginal breathing. The benefits don't stop there, though. Some research suggests that being in a cooler environment could be very healthy for you. A quick fix for chilling off? Nude yourself. Furthermore, you might be shocked to discover how remarkably freeing and powerful being nude can be!

Motives for Increasing Your Naked Time

My spouse and I used to make jokes about spending "naked" days at home early in our marriage. Please don't be too harsh on us; we were young at the time! It was still unusual to be nude. We used to make jokes about lounging around, cooking pancakes, spending entire days in our birthday suits, and doing other things that married couples do.

I can't help but giggle at our notion of married bliss when I look back. With four children and nearly ten years of marriage, our "naked" days don't look quite the same as they once did. But it's still a good idea to spend more time nude, regardless of your age, gender, or marital status.

Here are some justifications for enjoying more time spent in your birthday suit.

1. To feel more at ease in your own skin

Body image problems affect a lot of women, particularly after having kids. The majority of us are too familiar with the "tricks" that shield us from having to face our true selves in the nude. There's the complete avoidance of mirrors (don't look!), the insistence on installing only full-length mirrors (chest up, please!), and the hasty "towel wrap" (hurry, cover up!) following showers. Since I've completed them all, I completely understand.

However, making yourself spend more time in the nude forces you to acknowledge that this is your body. There is no need to feel embarrassed. Our bodies are amazing, no matter where you are in your health journey. They are essential to our survival and should be respected and cared for, not avoided at all costs.

Once you are at ease with the way your body appears, you might find it easier to accept the changes you need to make in order to develop a deeper sense of love for it.

2. To promote nursing

It could be easier for you to breastfeed if you spend more time topless. After nursing, letting your breasts air dry can aid in the healing of cracked nipples. Additionally, you might lessen your chance of developing mastitis. You can avoid infection by letting your breasts breathe naturally rather than cramming them into a tight bra with a milk pad that will soak up liquid and sit for a long time.

3. To promote closeness

Spending more time undressed together can inevitably lead to greater intimacy if you're married or in a relationship. While there might be merit in maintaining a sense of mystery in the bedroom, there's also merit in cuddling up close under the covers.

According to studies, oxytocin, or the "love" hormone, is promoted when a mother and child bond through breastfeeding and skin-to-skin contact. As it happens, adults experience the same thing. Keeping a physical connection fosters an emotional connection as well.

4. To encourage healthy vagina

It may be much healthier for you to expose your privates more frequently. There are types of underwear made of non-breathable fabric. These may increase a woman's risk of urinary tract infections (UTIs) and irritated skin. Although studies indicate that underwear made of synthetic fibers poses the highest risk of a UTI, even cotton can serve as a breeding ground for bacteria.

Especially if your vagina is irritated from shaving or frequent thong use, going pantless under a dress or at night can help your skin breathe and help the pH of your vagina naturally balance itself out.

5. To have a more restful night's sleep

Lowering your body temperature is one of the best strategies to improve your quality of sleep. Your body will be able to perform better while you sleep, in addition to having better quality sleep itself. When you're sleeping, your body goes through a lot of physical strain. It's burning off extra fat, generating new cells, and eliminating toxins. A study (Trusted Source) even discovered that sleeping in your undies at night can lower your body temperature and increase your body's metabolism and fat burning capacity. Being cozier at night is definitely not a bad thing, is it?

6. To feel content

Many of the things that people do in modern times have distanced us from our ancestral roots. However, it turns out that sometimes all we need to be happier and consequently healthier is to pare down to the essentials. According to one study, a person can improve their body image, self-esteem, and level of life satisfaction by just going nude more often. Reconnecting with nature in a very real way may actually improve your general happiness.

Chapter 2: Dry vagina's curse

Dryness in the Vagina

A painful symptom that many people may encounter at some point in their lives is vaginal dryness. This symptom may be brought on by certain medications, breastfeeding, or a drop in hormone levels. It is frequently connected to menopause. The cause of vaginal dryness usually determines the available treatment options.

Summary

What does dry vagina mean?

A painful symptom that lowers one's quality of life is vaginal dryness. It may hurt while you're sitting, working out, urinating, or having sex. Your vaginal lining is normally kept thick and elastic by a lubricating fluid. When the tissues in your vagina are thin, dry, and poorly moisturized, it can lead to vaginal dryness. This is uncomfortable, particularly when having sex.

Dry vagina can occur at any age. Women or those classified as female at birth (AFAB) are more likely to experience it during or after menopause, when estrogen levels start to drop. The hormone estrogen contributes to the health and hydration of your vaginal lining. You get thin, dry vaginal walls when your estrogen levels are low. Vaginal atrophy is a prevalent menopausal condition.

Is dry vaginal skin common?

Before menopause even, about 17% of individuals who were assigned female at birth (AFAB) and are between the ages of 18 and 50 reports experiencing vaginal dryness during sexual activity. After menopause, more than half report having dry vagina.

Potential Reasons

What could be the source of dry vagina?

Vaginal dryness frequently results from a drop in estrogen. This happens on its own as you get older or go through menopause. When your menstrual cycle ends and you are no longer able to conceive, you enter the menopause. Your vulva and vaginal skin and tissues become thinner and less elastic as your estrogen levels drop, and your vagina may become dry.

Vaginal dryness can also be brought on by certain medical disorders or their treatments. **Dry vagina can be caused by**:

- Childbirth and breastfeeding (chestfeeding).
- Birth control pills are one type of hormonal birth control.
- Chemotherapy and hormone therapy are two cancer treatments.

- Diabetes.
- Medications, such as antidepressants, antihistamines (for runny noses and itchy eyes), and anti-estrogens (for endometriosis or uterine fibroids).
- Your ovaries are removed (oophorectomy).
- Sjogren's syndrome: Autoimmune conditions that can make your entire body feel dry.
- Not experiencing sexual arousal.
- Using scented or perfumed washcloths, sprays, and soaps in your vagina or surrounding area.

Why does having sex make my vagina dry?

Sexual penetration is typically when vaginal dryness is most noticeable. Insufficient vaginal lubrication can result in pain and discomfort from the friction (or rubbing) that occurs during sexual activity. Make sure you're completely aroused before engaging in sexual activity. Try to unwind while having foreplay with your significant other. Water-based sexual lubricants can be beneficial as well. Regretfully, having uncomfortable sex can cause you to lose interest in having sex or intimacy with your partner. Talk to your partner about your symptom, no matter how embarrassing it may feel, so they can support you.

How does the vagina feel when it's dry?

Your vagina hurts and feels uncomfortable when you have dry vagina, especially during sex. Dry vaginas can also result in:

- Itching and burning.
- Bleeding following intercourse as a result of your vaginal wall tissues rupturing.
- Discomfort in your vulva.
- Yeast infections or recurring urinary tract infections (UTIs).
- Requiring more urination.
- Aversion to having sex.

Your vulvar region (external genitals) will become less moist as your vagina becomes less moist. This implies that wearing underwear and engaging in daily activities like walking or sitting might cause dryness or irritation.

Handling and Medical Care

How is the diagnosis of dry vagina made?

Medical professionals use a physical examination and your medical history to diagnose vaginal dryness. Your doctor will inquire about your symptoms and any medications you take in an effort to determine the cause. They could run the following examinations:

- Examine your pelvis to see the inside of your vagina, which could be red, dry, and thin.
- To find out if hormone levels or a medical condition are the cause of vaginal dryness, get a blood test.

In order to rule out other possible causes or look for indications of infection, your doctor might also test a sample of your vaginal discharge.

How is the dry vagina treated?

Vaginal dryness and its associated painful intercourse (dyspareunia) can be treated in a variety of ways.

Medications to treat dry vagina

Research indicates that a minimum of one in five females experience vaginal dryness, which is precisely what it sounds like. Numerous factors can contribute to it, including stress, insufficient foreplay, and antihistamine use, to mention a few. Fortunately, there are various treatment options available for it, ranging from using "things you have in your pantry" to obtaining necessary prescriptions from a physician.

1. **Lube, naturally.** Somehow, even after this website has been fervently supporting lubricant for almost forever, people still don't talk about it enough. Even if dryness isn't a problem, everyone

who engages in sexual activity ought to use lube. There are countless varieties of lubricant available, including silicone-based, water-based, vegan, and more. Your physician can provide suggestions if you're worried about allergies or need assistance selecting the one that suits you the best.

2. **Well, but**: Make an informed lubricant choice. You are unable to use oil-based lubricant while wearing latex condoms. Opt for a water- or silicon-based lubricant instead of oil-based lubricant, as the latter ruins latex condoms and makes them useless.

3. **Increase your foreplay**. In actuality, one can never have too much foreplay. Should there not be sufficient foreplay, someone might be somewhat dry and less lubricated "Brightman said. It's perfectly acceptable to ask your partners for a little more foreplay; there's nothing at all shameful or negative about wanting a little more attention to get things going in the bedroom. Try any of these, or whatever makes you happy, because you deserve it.

4. **Halt the hair removal process**. According to New York City ob-gyn Dr. Rebecca Brightman, pubic hair typically acts as a natural buffer to keep the skin on the vulva moist, and some women find

that shaving off their pubic hair causes dryness in the vagina and around the vulva.

5. **Moisturize the skin if you must remove your pubic hair**. If you find that shaving is leaving your skin dry, Brightman suggests using Aquaphor around the vulva instead of inside your vagina.

6. **No lubricant left?** Make use of these items in your pantry. According to Brightman, natural lubricants such as coconut oil, olive oil, and vegetable oil are all safe to use and can be applied directly to the vagina. "If someone finds that it's irritating they should stop," she stated. "But the vagina has a way of cleaning itself out in general, and I don't think anything like that would alter the [vaginal] pH so much that it'd be problematic."

7. **Change your allergy medication**. Vaginal dryness is a side effect of many allergy and cold medications that contain antihistamines. You can discuss other options that might be available to you with your doctor.

8. **Examine a hormone cream for topical use**. According to Brightman, women who are nursing or close to menopause frequently require a little extra assistance to relieve vaginal dryness. Your doctor might advise using a topical estrogen cream to help.

9. **Examine any skin issues**. According to Brightman, psoriasis and eczema can affect your vulva just like they can the rest of your body. Your dermatologist or gynecologist can check for skin conditions on the vagina and vulva and prescribe medication if necessary. Many creams for these conditions are only meant to be applied to specific body parts, so consult your doctor before slapping the steroid cream you use on your legs on your vulva.

10. **See a doctor if there is any itching, redness, or discharge**. According to Brightman, dryness is a common side effect of yeast infections. If this is the case, you can either get a diagnosis from your doctor or purchase an over-the-counter medication. Drugs function in your body by either acting as or substituting for estrogen. They can only be obtained with a prescription.

Low-dose estrogen tablets, creams, or rings: These drugs function by replenishing your body's supply of estrogen. Using an applicator, creams and tablets are injected straight into your vagina. The majority are prescribed to be taken once daily until relief is achieved, then once a week as needed. Your vagina is fitted with estrogen-containing rings, which are removed after up to three months.

Ospemifene, also known as Osphena, is a selective estrogen modulator (SERM) that is taken orally. It helps relieve painful sex related to vaginal atrophy and functions in your body similarly to estrogen.

Dehydroepiandrosterone (DHEA): This drug functions in your body similarly to estrogen. It's a vaginal suppository that relieves menopausal women's painful sex.

Discuss the risks and advantages of taking medication that contains estrogen or compounds that are similar to estrogen with your healthcare provider. For those who have had breast cancer or are at high risk of developing the disease, estrogen may not be safe.

Moisturizers and lubricants for dry vagina

Drug and grocery stores carry moisturizers and lubricants that can be bought without a prescription. They relieve sex-related pain by moistening and replenishing your vaginal tissue. Moisturizers designed for your face or bodies are not appropriate for use in your vagina.

Vaginal moisturizers: To maintain the health of your vaginal lining, apply vaginal moisturizers to the inside of your vagina every few days. Liquibeads and Replens Luvena are two examples.

Vaginal lubricants: Use lubricants right before a sexual encounter to reduce sex-related discomfort.

Two examples of water-based vaginal lubricants are KY Jelly and Astroglide. Additionally, there are lubricants based on silicone and oil.

Which foods make women more lubricated?

Research on particular foods you should eat to improve vaginal lubrication is lacking. Maintaining proper hydration and drinking water aid in the body's moisture retention.

How can a dry vagina be naturally treated?

Natural oils like coconut, grape seed, olive, vegetable, or sunflower oil may be a secure at-home treatment for dry vagina. Before having sex, apply natural oils externally as lubrication. Use only water-based lubricants if you are of childbearing age, as oil-based lubricants can harm condoms.

Some healthcare professionals advise having regular sex to help entice your vaginal tissues to moisten. Increasing the amount of foreplay time before sexual activity is another thing to try. Arousal and vaginal moisture are related. Before having sex, consider how you and your partner can enjoy each other more.

When to Make a Doctor's Appointment

When ought I to give my healthcare provider a call?

Although a dry vagina is typically not an indication of a serious medical condition, discussing it with your healthcare provider may make you feel awkward. However, there are numerous ways to treat this typical symptom. If you experience vaginal dryness, call your doctor.

Interferes with the things you do every day.

Impacts your relationship with your partner or your sexual life.

Doesn't improve with over-the-counter medication.

Is coupled with significant vaginal bleeding.

A message from Cleveland Clinic

One common symptom you'll probably encounter at some point in your life is vaginal dryness. Your vagina can become dry for a variety of reasons, including menopause or certain medications. This dry sensation may cause burning, itching, or soreness in your genitalia, as well as uncomfortable sex. If over-the-counter remedies don't relieve your vaginal dryness or if your symptoms get worse, see your healthcare provider.

Chapter 3: How to Enjoy Your Vagina

1. **Make use of condoms**. Although rubbers are well known for their ability to prevent sexually transmitted infections and pregnancy, a recent study discovered that condom use maintains the normal pH level of the vagina, which is necessary for the survival of beneficial bacteria like lactobacilli. And the reason this is so crucial is that those tiny bacteria guard against bacterial vaginosis, yeast infections, and urinary tract infections. In case you needed one more excuse to finish off.

2. **Go commando or put on cotton underwear**. Your vagina prefers cotton underwear when it comes to undergarments. For this reason, the majority of undergarments have a thin cotton fabric strip in the crotch. According to Yale University clinical professor of obstetrics, gynecology, and reproductive sciences Mary Jane Minkin, MD, it's the perfect way to cover your lady parts because it breathes and absorbs moisture. Additionally, Minkin advises going commando when you're just hanging around the house to let things out. Just remember to wear

underwear to the gym as you'll want an additional layer of protection from contaminated equipment.

3. **Solve the problem**. Kegel exercises are essential for building stronger pelvic floor muscles, which are necessary for bladder control as well as for stronger, mind-blowing orgasms. Make a note to yourself: Work out with Kegels every time. (Ingenious people are even developing a cool app to help with memory.)

4. **Adopt a Greek yogurt diet** According to Minkin, eating yogurt with live cultures as a snack increases the good bacteria in your vagina, which is great for preventing vaginal problems such as yeast infections. Just take care not to overindulge in the extremely sweet variety as that may increase your vulnerability to those infections.

5. **Attend your annual exam every year**. As Minkin points out, a visit to the doctor involves more than just sticking your tongue out when you're not pregnant and have no symptoms. New guidelines recommend against yearly pelvic exams in these situations. She says, I think it's important to talk about health problems with an annual exam. It's as important to use this time to discuss condom use, fertility, and any random questions you have about sex as it is to get tested for sexually

transmitted diseases. Therefore, discuss it with your doctor before you decide to alternate visits.

6. **Grease the machine**. Sometimes it seems like your vagina didn't get the memo that you were about to hit the sheets. However, it's completely normal—if you take certain medications, such as hormonal birth control, antidepressants, or antihistamines, vaginal dryness may affect you. Additionally, it may appear just before or after menopause. When this occurs, be sure to communicate with your partner so that they don't push past you before you're sufficiently lubricated. This can lead to abrasions and pain. To expedite the process and make sex even hotter, Minkin suggests simply using lube.

7. **Refrain from douching**. Do you feel like you could use some help keeping everything organized down there? You don't. According to Dena Harris, MD, a clinical assistant professor of obstetrics and gynecology at New York University, the vagina actually cleans itself. Furthermore, research indicates that the use of intravaginal hygiene products may raise your risk of STDs, infections, and pelvic inflammatory disease. Simply put, don't.

8. **Use caution when handling when cycling**. The cycling studio is one unexpected place you might

be endangering the health of your vagina. Regular riders may experience genital numbness, pain, and tingling while cycling, which is not a good thing. Actually, the majority of female cyclists in a study published in the Journal of Sexual Medicine reported having these symptoms. If you enjoy working out in cycling studios, consider wearing padded shorts and making the following form adjustments to prevent vaginal pain.

9. **Use caution when handling antibiotics**. Antibiotics pose a threat to the beneficial bacteria in your nether region. According to Minkin, those pills may eliminate some of the beneficial lactobacilli that maintain the health of your vagina. Naturally, you shouldn't refuse an antibiotic if it's necessary to fight an infection; instead, she advises loading up on probiotic Greek yogurt to minimize any harm.

10. **Pay attention to the sequence of sexual acts**. According to Minkin, be careful not to switch from anal to vaginal sex without changing the condom or thoroughly cleaning off beforehand. According to her, switching from the backdoor to the front can expose your vagina to a variety of bacteria and increase your risk of infection.

11. **Use soap with caution**. According to Minkin, as amazing as that scented body wash is, it has no

business being near your genitalia. To keep things clean around your vulva, you really just need to rinse with warm water. Soap can be extremely drying to the delicate skin in that area. But stick with a simple, mild, unscented soap if you just can't bring yourself to stop using soap, she advises.

Eight Causes of Vaginal Odor or Discomfort and How to Treat Them All as Per Experts

One of the most bothersome vaginal health problems is vaginal odor, along with painful vaginal dryness and the dreaded vaginal itching. It's reasonable to be concerned if you've ever noticed an unpleasant or unusual smell coming from your vagina, even though certain smells are perfectly normal.

The medical director of the Northwestern Medicine Center for Sexual Health and Menopause and author of Sex Rx: Hormones, Health, and Your Best Sex Ever, Lauren Streicher, M.D., says that your vagina shouldn't smell like roses and that many women mistakenly believe that something is wrong with them.

She clarifies, "There is a typical vaginal odor, but it shouldn't smell offensive." "A woman who grows up being taught that her genitalia are disgusting is more likely to detect a [bad] odor even in the absence of any abnormalities."

Thus, you're probably fine if your smell is the same as it has always been. If there's a funky smell coming from down there, though, and it seems unusual, don't disregard it. These are the main reasons for vaginal odor that you should be aware of.

Typical smells coming from the vagina

Certain vaginal smells are more prevalent than others. According to Christine Greves, M.D., a board-certified ob/gyn at the Winnie Palmer Hospital for Women and Babies, these are generally happy fairly often:

- A tart or acidic scent
- A smell like yeast
- A faintly sweet aroma
- A smell of metal
- A smell like ammonia
- A smell similar to body odor

Causes of Vaginal Odor

Certain causes of vaginal odor are expected in specific circumstances, while others are more reason for alarm.

Causes of vaginal odor that is typical

If you experience any of the causes of vaginal odor, don't panic. They are frequent and typically simple to fix.

It's sweaty down there.

According to board-certified obstetrician and gynecologist Kiarra King, M.D., F.A.C.O.G., body odor and a sweaty vagina are actually a "super common reason" for vaginal odor, despite the fact that it may sound straightforward. Dr. King says, "There's always going to be a higher propensity for sweating anywhere that there is a large number of hair follicles and sweat glands, which we find in the armpit and also in the pubic region with the pubic hair." Therefore, "where there is perspiration and moisture, and especially where there is hair that may retain moisture and bacteria, it's just the right combination for odor."

Treatment: Try to change into breathable cotton underwear as soon as possible after your workout, and throw away your panty liners. (Some brands, like these ones from Hanes, even have the ability to wick away sweat.) Since pubic hair can trap odor, especially in the warmer months, trimming it can also be beneficial.

You have an incorrect pH.

According to Dr. Streicher states that an imbalance in the normal flora in the vagina is the most common cause of vaginal odor. This imbalance causes irritation, a fishy smell, and thin to no vaginal discharge. Although these disagreeable bacteria can take over at any time, they are most likely to do so following a period or sexual encounter because semen and blood can alter your body's pH.

Yeast infections: what about them? They may give off a faint yeasty smell, but smell is rarely the primary issue. More often are itching and thick, white discharges.

Treatment: Antibiotics are required if it develops into a serious infection (also referred to as bacterial vaginosis; see below). However, you can often identify the issue before medication is necessary. RepHresh Vaginal Gel is recommended by Dr. Streicher to patients as a way to balance the pH in your vagina. After two treatments, you should see a significant improvement, she says. If not, it's time to give your doctor a call and most likely obtain a prescription.

Unusual reasons for vaginal odor

A visit to the doctor is usually necessary to address these causes of vaginal odor.

Lack of continence

"The first thing to determine when discussing vaginal odor is if it is actually coming from the vagina or if it is actually a genital odor." Dr. Streicher states. (Remember that your vulva, or external genitals, is everything that surrounds your vagina, which is located inside your body.) "A lot of women experience incontinence." Women frequently have very little leakage that they are unaware of—they typically only notice the odor.

Treatment: Showering and changing clothes should take care of this problem as it is external in nature (urine hanging around your genitals or underwear). However, if you frequently struggle to get to the bathroom in time, do let your doctor know. Medication and other therapies are available that may be helpful.

You're keeping a tampon that you forgot.

Although it may sound absurd, many women, according to Dr. Streicher, forget to remove their tampon after inserting one. It's possible that you put one in "just in case" even though your period was about to end and forgot about it because it was the end of the month. You could have removed the first tampon and carelessly put in a new one. According to Dr. Streicher, the smell will be quite strong if it has been inside for a while.

Treatment: Yes, that's right—you have to remove the tampon. You can try to remove it yourself, or your doctor can do it with ease: Place two fingers deep into your vagina while lying flat on your back. According to Dr. Streicher, Women can probably get it out themselves, but most of the time they don't even know it's there.

The disease caused by bacteria

The most common form of vaginitis, or inflammation of the vagina, is bacterial vaginosis (BV), which most women will encounter at some point in their lives, according to Jerome Chelliah, M.D., board-certified ob/gyn at HerMD. He states that "BV is caused by a change in the vaginal microbiome," explaining that this occurs when an excess of anaerobic bacteria replaces the lactobacilli, the predominant vaginal bacteria, changing the pH of the vagina. He goes on to say, this pH shift is the cause of BV symptoms, such as vaginal discharge, odor, and irritation.

Sexual stimulation, douching, and the use of specific fragrances and detergents can alter the pH of the vagina and aggravate bacterial vaginosis symptoms.

Treatment: A device known as a wet mount will be used by your physician to diagnose your BV. For this kind of test, a vaginal sample is taken and examined under a microscope. Dr. Chelliah says you will be prescribed a course of antibiotics, like metronidazole or clindamycin, if abnormal cells are found. He says that there are other medications that could be used if those don't seem to be helping.

The Trichomonas Infection

According to Dr. King, infections are yet another extremely typical source of vaginal odor. Furthermore, trichomoniasis is an infection that also "causes an odor that's pretty distinctive for most people," though bacterial vaginosis is frequently the primary offender. Though it can be spread that way, bacterial vaginosis is not officially classified as a sexually transmitted infection (STI), but trichomoniasis is. According to Dr. King It may result in a thin, watery-gray discharge, there may be some irritation or itching, and people may describe the smell as fishy or foul from the vaginal or vulvar area."

Treatment: According to Dr. King, trichomoniasis is an infection that must be cleared with a course of prescription antibiotics in order to alleviate symptoms. This prescription can be obtained from your gynecologist, family physician, internal medicine physician, or even an emergency room physician, depending on who makes the diagnosis.

It's important to note that the Centers for Disease Control and Prevention (CDC) recommends that healthcare professionals counsel patients suffering from trichomoniasis infections to refrain from having sex until after treatment for themselves and their partner(s) has been completed and any symptoms have subsided. People with trichomoniasis should also be tested for syphilis, gonorrhea, Chlamydia, HIV, and other STIs.

Uncommon Reasons for Vaginal Odor

Although these possible causes of vaginal odor are uncommon, physicians advise discussing them just in case.

Cervical cancer

Cancer of the uterine cervix, the opening to the uterus, is known as cervical cancer. Additionally, it occasionally causes vaginal odor. According to Dr. Chelliah, it's the fourth most common cancer in women worldwide and frequently goes undiagnosed since so many people don't show any symptoms. Therefore, routine screening with a Pap smear, or Pap test, is crucial for preventing cancer, he says. "A person may have symptoms like vaginal bleeding (especially after sex), vaginal discharge, and possibly vaginal odor if cervical cancer advances."

Although that may seem frightening, you shouldn't panic just yet because vaginal odor isn't typically a sign of cervical cancer.

Treatment: See your doctor for an evaluation if you're concerned that your symptoms could indicate cervical cancer. They will check you out and perform a pap smear. If abnormal cells are found, a colposcopy, or procedure to examine the cervix under a special microscope, is carried out, Dr. Chelliah states. "A biopsy, or small sample of tissue taken during a colposcopy, is sent to the laboratory for additional analysis and cervical cancer diagnosis."

Depending on how far the cancer has progressed, your doctor and I will decide on the best course of action if the lab results reveal cervical cancer. According to Dr. Chelliah, this may involve radiation, chemotherapy, or surgery.

Rectovaginal Fistula

According to Dr. Greves, a rectovaginal fistula is an abnormal connection between the vagina and the rectum or anus. She claims that as a result, the contents of your bowel can seep into the vagina through that opening. Dr. Greves remarks, "You're basically having poop inside the vagina." "It has an awful odor."

This will frequently result in an odd discharge and a smell similar to rotten meat or sewer, according to her.

Treatment: According to Dr. Greves, treatment options include surgery to seal the opening and antibiotics if there is an infection surrounding the fistula. In either case, a medical professional's assistance is required to solve the issue.

What is the duration of vaginal odor?

According to Dr. Greves, it really depends on the underlying cause and what you do about it. For instance, until they are treated, trichomoniasis and BV will continue to produce an unpleasant smell. She notes, something like sweat can also come back and cause an odor again.

But according to Dr. Greves, if you're being treated for an odor-causing illness, the smell ought to go away in a few days to a week.

How does pregnancy affect the smell of the vagina?

According to Dr. Greves, there are numerous hormonal changes that occur during pregnancy, including variations in prolactin, progesterone, and estrogen levels. According to her, that can affect your vaginal pH and change your vaginal odor.

Pregnancy also increases the likelihood of vaginal inflammation, or vaginitis. Dr. Greves advises, "If it smells fishy, mention it to your healthcare provider," noting that BV may be the cause.

Methods for avoiding vaginal odor

Although your vagina doesn't have to smell like a flower arrangement, there are methods to stop vaginal odor before it starts if you are sensitive to certain scents.

Apply a gentle cleanser.

Dr. King advises against using anything in the vagina and instead applying a light, fragrance-free soap (or even just water) externally on the vulva area. According to Dr. King, you should be cautious about the products you use down there and make sure you are "cleaning between the folds of the labia to remove any buildup."

Refrain from douching

Douching "will disrupt your pH" and "leads to a vicious cycle" of vaginal odor problems, according to Dr. King, so using products intended to flush or cleanse your vagina can actually worsen the smell of your vagina even though they claim to do the opposite. "It is unnecessary to take any action that could potentially disturb the vaginal flora and the normal pH environment of the vagina as the vagina is self-cleaning," says Dr. King. Basically, it's better to let your body heal itself and leave the specialty cleansers and douches on the shelf.

Consume a well-rounded diet.

"Food can affect vaginal odor, according to research," Dr. Chelliah adds. Unfortunately, some of your favorites can change the scent of your vagina, including coffee, onions, garlic, strong spices, dairy, and too much meat or alcohol.

Remain hydrated.

Your urine may smell strongly of ammonia due to dehydration, and this peculiar odor may linger for a while. Getting enough water helps to dilute waste, this improves the smell of both your poop and your pants.

Put on airy, light clothing.

Funk is more likely to occur when clothing is too tight because more heat and moisture are trapped in and around the vulva. Dr. King advises against dressing too tight or wearing cotton underwear because doing so creates a "setup" for odor caused by perspiration and bacterial growth.

When to consult a physician for vaginal odor

In general, it's a good idea to visit a healthcare professional if an odd smell continues and is accompanied by other symptoms like pain, burning, itching, or an odd discharge. According to Dr. King, any unusual or uncomfortable discharge or odor "certainly should be evaluated and checked out."

Chapter 4: Kegel Exercises

Kegel Exercises

Your pelvic floor muscles can become stronger with Kegel exercises. The group of muscles in your pelvic floor that you use to halt the flow of urine. By making these muscles stronger, you can avoid inadvertently passing gas or poop or leaking urine. It offers advantages for both vaginal and penile users.

A Kegel exercise: what is it?

Your pelvic floor muscles can be strengthened with kegel exercises, also known as pelvic floor exercises. The muscles of your pelvic floor support the organs in your pelvis, including the bladder, bowel, and vagina. Your pelvic floor muscles help with sex, urination, and other body functions while also supporting the position of your organs. Kegel exercises strengthen your pelvic floor muscles by first tightening and then relaxing them.

Kegel exercises can assist with problems like:
- Urine leakage or incontinence.
- Urge incontinence, or the sudden need to urinate.
- Defecation (leaking of feces).

Pelvic organ prolapse refers to the sagging or bulging of the pelvic organs into the vagina.

Kegel exercises can also help you have better orgasms and enhance your sexual health. Kegel exercises are beneficial for both men and women who were assigned male or female at birth (AMAB and AFAB, respectively).

What is the real purpose of Kegel exercises?

Your pelvic floor muscles will stay "fit" if you perform Kegel exercises. Kegel exercises are a good method to maintain the strength of your pelvic floor muscles, just as lifting weights can help strengthen other muscles in your body. Kegel exercises can help you maintain stronger pelvic muscles and improve control over your bowel and bladder movements.

It's possible to inadvertently pass gas or leak poop and urine due to weak pelvic floor muscles. The muscles that support your pelvic floor may weaken as you age or as a result of pregnancy, childbirth, or surgery.

Does anyone need to perform Kegel exercises?

Anything that strains your pelvic floor muscles may weaken them and reduce their ability to support your pelvic organs. Your pelvic floor muscles may become weak due to specific medical conditions or life events. Among these circumstances and occurrences are:

Maternity

- Birthing, including cesarean sections.
- Being overweight (BMI greater than 25) or obese (body mass index, or BMI, greater than 30).
- Surgery pertaining to your pelvis.

Growing older.

As you age, the muscles in your rectum, anus, and pelvic floor naturally deteriorate.

Persistent coughing or excessive straining when passing gas (constipation).

Workouts (particularly sprinting, jumping, and lifting big weights).

Kegel exercises aren't appropriate for everyone, though. Overdoing Kegel exercises or performing Kegels when not necessary can lead to overly tight or tense muscles.

Exercises for Kegels and pregnancy

Doing Kegel exercises while pregnant may make delivery easier for expectant mothers. This is because, during labor and delivery, it might provide you more control over your pelvic muscles. It can also be beneficial for:

- Bladder management.
- Enhancing the fetal weight-bearing muscles' strength.
- Leakage of urine or urinary incontinence.
- Pushing when giving birth vaginally.
- Healing of the perineal after delivery.

How can I locate my muscles in my pelvic floor?
Try stopping the flow of your urine while seated on the toilet to identify your pelvic floor muscles. Do not stop until you have a sense of how it feels; otherwise, you run the risk of becoming infected. It's also possible to picture yourself attempting to stop yourself from passing gas.

Another option is to put your finger inside your vagina and squeeze the surrounding muscles. Your finger should be under pressure. The muscles that you strengthen during Kegel exercises are the same ones that you feel "lifting" when you perform these exercises.

Comparing your pelvic floor to a claw vending machine game you may have played as a kid could be useful. A metal claw opens up and extends downward in a claw machine game. When it opens, it takes up a ball, toy, or piece of candy before shutting. The claw returns to its initial position and remains closed after it has closed around your prize. The way the claw closes and draws upward is almost exactly like a Kegel.

How are Kegel exercises performed?

When you perform Kegel exercises, your pelvic floor muscles are lifted, held, and then relaxed. Begin by performing a small number of Kegels at a time, and then progressively increase the duration and quantity of Kegels performed in each "session" (or set). At least two or three sets of these exercises should be done each day.

An example of a Kegel schedule

Always keep in mind that you will gradually increase the intensity of your Kegel exercises. You won't be able to hold your Kegel for more than five or ten seconds at first. Also, you cannot anticipate outcomes immediately.

Here's an example of how to start Kegel exercises:

Locate your pelvic floor muscles first (by following the above steps).

For the first three seconds, tense your pelvic floor muscles, and then release the tension for another three seconds. One Kegel, that is.

Try to do this ten times over. If ten seems too much, start with five and work your way up to **We refer to this as a set.**

Perform a morning set and a nighttime set.

Try raising these numbers as you get stronger. For instance, hold your Kegels for five seconds each time, as opposed to three seconds of holding and three seconds of relaxing.

Next, if it isn't already the case, raise the quantity of Kegels to ten consecutive ones.

Lastly, up the frequency of these exercises from twice daily to three times daily.

Eventually, you should be able to do three sets of Kegels a day, holding and relaxing for five seconds between each set.

To achieve Kegels, how hard should I squeeze?

To feel Kegels working, you must squeeze or tighten sufficiently. On the other hand, take care not to compress or strain your back, stomach, buttocks, or inner thighs. If you are squeezing these muscles, the exercise is not being performed correctly.

Additionally, you shouldn't hold your breath by squeezing too hard. Breathe normally during the Kegel exercises. Counting aloud can assist you in keeping your regular breathing pattern.

Is standing or sitting better for Kegel exercises?

The Kegel exercises can be performed in a sitting or standing position. You might want to start off doing these exercises while lying down if your pelvic muscles are weak

For what amount of time is a Kegel held correctly?

Start with a limited number of Kegel exercises that are manageable for you. Take five Kegel exercises, for instance, and hold each one for three seconds twice a day. Increase these numbers gradually as your strength and endurance improve. Ideally, you should be able to hold the Kegels for five seconds and then release your muscles for the same amount of time. At least twice or three times a day, repeat this up to ten times.

Which Kegel exercise is the best?

The "best" Kegel exercise doesn't really exist. All Kegel exercises are useful when done properly. You may do kegel exercises in a sitting, standing, or laying down position. Select the option that most comfortably suits you. You should concentrate on lifting and squeezing in all positions, as if using your pelvic floor to pick up an object.

Why am I finding it difficult to perform Kegel exercises?

Your healthcare provider may recommend biofeedback training and electric stimulation of your pelvic floor muscles if you are having difficulty performing Kegel exercises.

A medical professional inserts a probe into your vagina during biofeedback. You are asked to perform a Kegel by your provider. A monitor indicates whether you are contracting the right muscles.

The sensation of a Kegel exercise is replicated by electrical stimulation. Your healthcare provider will apply a tiny electric current to your pelvic floor muscles during electrical stimulation. Your muscles then squeeze in response to the current.

If you're having trouble performing Kegels or aren't sure if you're using the correct muscles, don't be afraid to speak with a healthcare professional. They are available to assist you.

Kegel balls: what are they?

Kegel balls are unique devices that are worn within the vagina. These primarily round or circular devices, sometimes referred to as Kegel exercisers, aid in toning your pelvic floor muscles. Kegel balls are inserted into your vagina in a similar manner to how a tampon is. While you carry on with your regular activities, the Kegel ball is held in place by the muscles of your pelvic floor. You begin by wearing a Kegel ball for a short while each day, and you progressively extend its use.

How much time does it take to see results?

After six to eight weeks, you should start to notice results. The degree of muscle weakness and the consistency with which you perform Kegel exercises determine how long it takes to see results.

Does Kegel exercise apply to men?

Kegel exercise is beneficial for men and people AMAB with specific medical and sexual health issues. Men's Kegel exercises or individuals AMAB can:

Assist in reducing incontinence (based on the cause).

Assist in controlling swelling and pain in the prostate that arises from benign prostatic hyperplasia (BPH) and prostatitis.

Aid in erections and ejaculation to enhance sexual pleasure.

A message from Cleveland Clinic

Kegel exercises are helpful exercises to strengthen your muscles in your pelvic floor. There are numerous causes of weak pelvic floors. Signs of a weak pelvic floor include leaking urine or feces and feeling the urge to urinate when not necessary. Work your way up to executing Kegels multiple times a day. Never hesitate to seek assistance from a healthcare professional if you have questions

about Kegel exercises or are unsure if you are
performing them correctly.

Chapter 5: The Ideal vagina

Which vaginal types are there?
Shape, color, and size naturally vary in the vulva and its external structures. Although there are no particular varieties of vagina, each person's vagina will have unique qualities.

The majority of people ponder, "Am I normal?" when it comes to anything having to do with their bodies and sexual and reproductive health. There is a large range of healthy forms, sizes, and colors associated with the vagina.

This book explains the various kinds of vaginas, their variations, and when to visit a physician.

Is this normal for my vagina?
An ordinary vagina does not exist. The vulva, or outer portion, and the vagina, or internal female genitalia, vary from person to person.

While vaginas can vary greatly, most people's have a similar shape overall. Reliable Source with regard to:

Length, width, shape, quantity, color, discharge, and odor of pubic hair, or lips

Forms
The visible, external portion of the genitalia is typically meant when someone refers to the

vagina. The vulva is the anatomical term for this region.

Numerous structures make up the vulva, including the inner and outer lips, or labia majora and minora. These are the skin folds that encircle the urethral and vaginal openings.

The appearance of the vulva can differ greatly depending on the dimensions and form of the external structures. Studies that demonstrate a wide range of vulva morphologies have demonstrated this.

Any variation in this shape or size is almost never reason for alarm. Images of the external female genitalia can be found online to view this great range of forms.

Considering this diversity, some vulva traits that are common include:

Outer Lip

Some people have longer labia majora, or the vulva's outer lips. The skin may appear thin and the lips may drop, or they may be thick and swollen.

Generally speaking, the outer lips are smoother and do not fold as much as the inner lips.

Some people have outer lips that nearly completely conceal their inner lips and clitoris. In certain cases, some of the inner lips above may be visible as the outer lips curve and meet at the ends.

Short outer lips might not meet and might make the inner lips stand out more.

Inner Lips

The labia minora, or inner lips, are usually visible. They could protrude in other ways or dangle beneath the outer lips.

You might have one longer inner lip than the other. In general, asymmetry in the labia does not warrant concern.

Some people may have short lips on the inside that are hidden by full lips. In some, the length of the inner and outer lips is the same.

The clitoral hood, which covers the clitoris, may be seen if the outer and inner lips are small and near the inner thighs.

Healthy vulvas come in a wide range of sizes and shapes; these are just a few potential shape variations.

Within The Vagina

The vagina's interior resembles a long tube with folds that allow it to expand and contract.

According to imaging studies, most vaginas are wider near the cervix and narrower toward the vaginal opening. This typically takes the form of a "V," though the width varies at its widest point.

After delivery, their vagina may appear looser or wider. This occurs as a result of the vaginal tissues expanding to allow the baby to pass through the birth canal. The vagina may shrink back to its pre-pregnancy size or continue to enlarge slightly.

The majority of research on vaginal anatomy focuses on white females. However, there may be additional internal and external variations between white female genitalia and those of black or other non-white ethnicities.

The hymen

In the majority of females, the vaginal opening is partially covered by the hymen, a thin membrane. The hymen, which some liken to a scrunch hairstyle, is shielded from harm by the labia.

The elasticity and shape of hymens vary widely, and they can alter with age or during pregnancy.

The vagina may occasionally be completely covered by the hymen. As a result, complications may arise since the body may be unable to expel menstrual blood.

It's a myth that a person's hymen can reveal whether or not they are a virgin. Some people may bleed during their first sex, but this is not always the case. Tears in the hymen might be one cause of this.

Dimensions

To make room for a tampon, finger, or penis, for example, the vagina can enlarge or shorten. It elongates and stretches to accomplish this. The uterus and cervix are also moved upward by this.

The average vaginal length is slightly less than 4 inches, although this varies depending on the individual. MRI scans were utilized in this study to measure the vaginal length, width, and angles of the participants.

Nonetheless, the majority of studies indicate that some people's vaginas measure as much as 7 to 7.5 inches.

Researchers use the average length of the anterior (near the bladder) and posterior (near the rectum) vaginal walls to calculate the length of a vagina. The duration can, however, differ greatly.

Vibrance

Skin tones are naturally diverse, even in vulva skin.

The vulva's color could be:

- Reddish-pink,
- wine-colored

Blood flow can also have an impact on color. Blood flow increases and the vulva may appear purplish during arousal.

Some individuals observe changes in color when they experience specific medical conditions. For instance, a yeast infection could make the vulva look red or purple.

Hair

It is possible that pubic hair shields the genitalia from bacterial infections. Given that it typically develops during puberty, it may also be a sign of sexual maturity.

Everybody has different amounts, colors, and textures of pubic hair.

Vaginal type

Vaginas can have a variety of sizes, shapes, and colors. There is a lot of diversity, and men have different tastes. Here are the top five vaginal types that most appeal to men.

1. **The vaginal bone head**: It is likely that your vagina is narrow and bony if you are small in stature. Men adore it because it allows for a slightly tighter fit, guaranteeing an amazing experience. Because they never have to worry about being big enough, they also greatly boost men's confidence.

2. **The fatty lip vagina**: Popular among men, the fatty lip vagina is incredibly soft. They seem more approachable and simpler to locate for penetration.

Additionally uncommon in a fatty lip vagina are ingrown hairs.

3. **The virginal vagina**: If you have a tight virginal vagina, your partner will be pleased. It's possible that your vagina's walls are closing in due to their extreme tightness. Great stimulation and sex are provided by the snug fit. Men will believe that your vagina was made just for them if it fits them closely.

4. **The experienced, always-ready vagina**: This type of vagina draws men in because of her experience and constant readiness. Men are always satisfied with its perfect texture and tightness.

5. **Peek-a-boo vagina**: This type of vagina indicates that your clitoris is about to give you the ideal hint. You may only need to be touched or tickled on the clitoris for you to become attracted. Men adore the orgasms you get from these because they let them know they are doing a great job at what they do.

Note: Studies have shown that early onset of puberty in children, including pubic hair growth, may indicate a higher risk of polycystic ovarian syndrome (PCOS).

Release

The secretions and discharge from the vagina support the health of the vaginal tissues.

Some monitor their fertility by analyzing the color and consistency of their discharge. For instance, a few days prior to ovulation, an increase in discharge typically takes place.

Vaginal discharge changes may be a sign of an infection that requires medical intervention. If someone has a discharge that is green, gray, or smells bad, they should visit a doctor.

Gushing blood

Menstrual blood has an exit point in the vagina. A person may lose different amounts of blood during different periods. While some people often only have light spots, others frequently experience severe bleeding.

A doctor should be consulted by anyone whose menstrual flow frequently soaks pads or causes them to feel lightheaded or breathless. Anemia may arise from a heavy menstrual flow, which can also interfere with everyday activities. It might also be an indication of a medical issue that requires attention.

In certain situations, a physician might recommend birth control tablets to help control excessive menstrual flow.

Aroma

Odor-causing bacteria and yeasts are found in the vagina naturally. The aroma can range from metallic to sweet.

Vaginal odor can be influenced by a person's menstrual cycle, general health, and the natural flora of the vagina.

Variations in the smell of the vagina are usually not alarming. Nevertheless, an unpleasant odor may be a sign of a trichomoniasis or bacterial vaginosis infection.

When to visit a doctor anyone experiencing issues with their vulva or vagina should consult a physician

Typical worries include the following:

- Unusual outburst
- Strange odor and a shift in the labial tissues' color
- Severe bleeding, discomfort during intercourse, pelvic pain, and delayed menstruation around puberty
- Certain individuals have birth defects that may need to be surgically corrected.

For instance, some people have a wall across or down the vagina, which is known as a vaginal septum. There are two portions of the vagina due to the wall. It may cause issues during sex and have an impact on menstruation. This can be fixed with surgery.

Other odd characteristics that someone might be born with include:

- Vaginal agenesis, in which the vagina ceases to develop prior to childbirth, resulting in a shorter vagina or possibly none at all.
- A micro perforated hymen, where the hymen almost covers the vagina, making it difficult to remove a tampon; an imperforate hymen, where the hymen blocks the opening to the vagina, preventing menstrual blood from leaving the body; a septate hymen, where a band of extra tissue in the hymen divides the vaginal opening in two

This might go unnoticed until a person begins their menstrual cycle or engages in sexual activity.

Summary

The vagina and vulva can play many roles, from childbirth to menstrual flow and sexual pleasure.

The majority of shape, size, and color differences are beneficial. Nonetheless, a person should see a doctor if they have any concerns regarding their vulva or vagina.

Chapter 6: Vaginal infections that attack

A vaginal infection may occasionally show no symptoms at all. However, there are other instances when itching, changes in the color or volume of discharge, and pain when urinating are typical signs of an infection.

The term "vaginalitis" describes a number of distinct illnesses that can inflame or infect your vagina. Inflammation of the vulva, the external portion of your genitalia, as well as the vagina are both referred to by the similar umbrella term vulvovaginitis.

Vaginal infections are fairly common and have a wide range of potential causes. Actually, according to the American College of Obstetricians and Gynecologists, vaginal infections may occur in as many as one-third of vaginal users at some point in their lives.

Although these infections can occur at any time, they are most common from the late teens to the early 40s, which is when you are fertile.

Without engaging in any kind of sexual activity, including penetrative sex, one can still get a vaginal infection. Put another way, while some forms of sexual activity may occasionally contribute, vaginitis is not the same as a sexually transmitted infection (STI); further information on this point is provided below.

Continue reading to find out more about the common forms of vaginitis, as well as information on how to treat and relieve symptoms, causes, and remedies.

Vaginal infection types

Many of the symptoms of vaginal infections are similar, which can make it challenging to diagnose the condition accurately.

That said, there are a few distinct symptoms associated with each type of infection:

Bacteria-causing illness (BV). Thin grayish-white, greenish, or yellow discharge is frequently the result of BV. There may be a fishy smell to this discharge, and it usually gets stronger after penetrating vaginal sex. Perhaps there won't be much itching.

Infections with yeast. They frequently involve burning, soreness, and vaginal and vulva itching. Swelling in the labia, or the skin folds outside of the vagina, is another symptom of yeast infections. Any discharge will typically have a texture similar to cottage cheese and be lumpy and white in appearance.

Trichomoniasis. Usually, this infection results in both fishy-smelling vagina and itching. You may experience vaginal and vulva swelling, irritation, and inflammation in addition to a greenish-yellow, foamy discharge. Additional signs and symptoms of trichomoniasis include lower abdominal pain, burning sensations during urination, and pain during vaginal sex.

Vaginitis with Atrophy. Although this isn't technically an infection, it may raise your risk of getting UTIs and vaginal infections. Atrophic vaginitis can present with symptoms such as burning, itching, dryness, and changes in discharge in the vagina that are similar to those of other infections.

Signs and symptoms

Not all vaginal infections result in obvious symptoms.

If you do experience symptoms, you'll probably experience some of the following typical ones:

- Burning and itching in the vagina
- Discomfort and soreness in the vaginal area redness, flushing, or swelling of the skin surrounding the vulva
- A shift in the volume of discharge from the vagina

- Pain or burning when urinating; a change in the color of vaginal discharge; pain during penetrative vaginal sex
- Vaginal Spotting or Bleeding

You may be experiencing one or more of the above symptoms. It's critical to get in touch with a healthcare provider for a diagnosis and treatment if your symptoms worsen or don't go away after a few days.

Some of these symptoms may also be present in the event that you have a urinary tract infection (UTI), particularly a burning or painful feeling when urinating. This is how a UTI is identified.

How are infections of the vagina treated?

The cause of a vaginal infection will determine how it is treated.

A medical professional may recommend:

- Antifungal creams or suppositories to treat a yeast infection;
- Metronidazole (in tablet, cream, or gel form) or clindamycin (in cream or gel form) to treat a bacterial infection.
- Additionally, you can buy medicines for yeast infections without a prescription at your neighborhood drugstore or pharmacy, but if the infection doesn't go away or keeps coming back, you should see a doctor.

- Take tablets of metronidazole or tinidazole to treat trichomoniasis.
- Tablets or creams containing estrogen to help treat atrophic vaginitis-related severe vaginal dryness and irritation
- Healthcare providers typically advise against using irritants like douches, scented tampons or pads, and strong or perfumed soap.

Why do vaginal infections occur?

- To put it simply, vaginal infections typically occur when something alters the normal balance of yeast and bacteria in your vagina.
- By type of infection, the following are the common causes of vaginal infections:
- Infections caused by bacteria. BV is caused by an overabundance of specific naturally occurring bacteria in your vagina. Although hand-to-genital, oral, and penetrative vaginal sex are not classified as sexually transmitted infections (STIs), they can cause an overgrowth of bacteria and raise your risk of contracting bacterial vaginosis (BV).
- Infections with yeast. A fungus known as Candida albicans is typically the cause of yeast infections. Antibiotics, hormonal fluctuations, weakened immune systems,

and stress are just a few of the variables that can lower the quantity of antifungal bacteria in your vagina and cause an overabundance of yeast. A yeast infection may manifest as symptoms of this overgrowth.

- Trichomoniasis. This infection is brought on by the protozoan parasite Trichomonas vaginalis. The majority of cases of trichomoniasis are caused by anal, oral, or vaginal sex without the use of an internal or external condom. However, sharing bath water can also spread the infection. Additional uncommon (but feasible) means of transmission include shared towels or damp clothing, pools, and moist toilet seats.

- Atrophy of the vagina. This disorder usually appears after menopause, but it can also occur during nursing or at any other time when your estrogen levels fall. Vaginal thinning and dryness can result from low hormone levels, and this can exacerbate vaginal inflammation.

- Sagging. It may seem like a good idea to keep your vagina clean to flush it with a solution of water and vinegar, baking soda, iodine, or other antiseptic ingredients. Actually, though, your vagina can maintain cleanliness on its own. In fact, by reducing the amount of good bacteria in your vagina, this practice increases your risk of infection.

- Body wash, perfume, and soap. The natural pH of your vagina can also be upset by cleaning it with soap and body wash or misting it with perfume. Rinsing your vulva and vagina with plain water is perfectly OK, but using any other product or fragrance can kill good bacteria and increase the risk of infection.

- Spermicidal birth control. This birth control method may be supplied as a gel, film, or suppository. It dissolves when inserted directly into the vagina, killing sperm and preventing unintended pregnancy. Spermicidal may be effective for certain individuals, but they also increase the risk of vaginal infections and can cause irritation and inflammation in the vagina.

- Clothing that is synthetic or too tight. Tights and undergarments that are unable to "breathe" can irritate the vagina by holding in moisture and restricting airflow, increasing the risk of infections. Similar results can be obtained from wearing extremely tight underwear or from leaving wet underwear on after a swim or workout.

- Both fabric softener and detergent. Have you experienced symptoms soon after switching laundry detergents? Yeast infections and vaginal pH can both be impacted by scented fabric softener and detergent.

A medical practitioner may occasionally be unable to identify the source of your vaginal infection. We refer to this illness as nonspecific vulvovaginitis. Although vaginal haves of any age can experience it, young people who have not yet reached puberty are more likely to experience it.

How are infections of the vagina identified?

A medical professional can assist in the diagnosis of a vaginal infection.

To assist in determining whether you have a yeast infection (BV), you can also use an at-home vaginal pH test, which is available online and in certain pharmacies.

A physician or other healthcare professional may question you if you frequently get vaginal infections, particularly of the same kind, in order to help diagnose the infection and determine its cause.

One may inquire:

Concerning your sexual partners; whether you use condoms during vaginal sex; your medical history, including any history of vaginal infections; whether you douche or wash your vagina with soap; and whether you use scented period products.

Regarding other medical conditions' symptoms

In addition, depending on your symptoms, they could

Examine the pelvis to check for any irritation or inflammation.

Gather a vaginal discharge sample to submit for examination.

Test for STIs like gonorrhea or Chlamydia by swabbing your cervix.

Collect a urine sample for STI detection.

Between bacterial vaginosis and yeast infection

Some symptoms of both BV and yeast infections are similar, making it easy to confuse the two.

When it comes to receiving the appropriate care, this may present an issue. OTC medications can be used to treat yeast infections, negating the need for medical attention from a physician. Conversely, BV frequently necessitates the use of prescription-only antibiotics for treatment.

82

These DIY cures might lessen the symptoms of BV.

You can distinguish between the two with this chart.

	Bacterial vaginosis	Yeast infection
Odor	often causes a fish-like smell, especially after vaginal sex	usually doesn't cause an odor
Discharge texture	thin and watery, sometimes foamy	thick and clumpy
Discharge color	grayish or greenish	white
Vulva appearance	you may not notice any change	inflamed, reddish, or lighter or darker in color, often with a white

		coating around the outside of your vagina
Itching and burning	not necessarily, though you might notice itching if you have more discharge	very common, especially during urination
Treatment	antibiotics	often clears up with OTC treatment

How can vaginal infections be avoided?

While it is not possible to prevent every vaginal infection, following advice can lessen your risk of getting one:

Steer clear of scented tampons, pads, and liners when using period products.

Steer clear of scented sprays or perfumes in your vagina, douching, and vaginal deodorants.

Because scented body washes and bubble baths can alter the pH of the vagina, only take plain water baths. Are you trying to find a vaginal cleaner? Look through our guide.

Sex toys should be washed in accordance with their care guidelines after each use. Prevent sharing sex toys by cleaning them first.

Put on cotton underwear or underwear with a cotton crotch to enhance ventilation and lessen irritation and inflammation in the vagina. Alternate your underwear after working out, or at least once a day.

Wear pantyhose, tights, leggings, and exercise pants with a cotton crotch instead.

To help prevent excess moisture, change out of your swimsuits and damp exercise gear as soon as possible.

Forget the scented fabric softener and use an unscented or sensitive skin detergent instead.

Even though vaginal infections are not regarded as sexually transmitted infections, using condoms during intercourse can help reduce your risk of getting one.

Recall that condoms help prevent changes in vaginal pH that could upset the delicate balance of bacteria in your vagina in addition to providing protection against STIs.

When selecting and applying condoms, bear the following in mind:

- Do not use flavored condoms for sex in the vagina.
- Spermicidal or pre-lubricated condoms may also irritate.
- After anal intercourse, always use a fresh condom for vaginal penetration.

Searching for a different kind or brand of condom? You have many choices in this situation.

- When is the right time to visit a physician or other healthcare provider?
- Certain vaginal infections may go away on their own without the need for medical attention, particularly if you use over-the-counter or home remedies to hasten the infection's progression.

Nevertheless, infections may not always get better on their own. You should schedule a visit with your physician or other healthcare provider if you:

- Have never had a vaginal infection previously, or if you have, your symptoms are new or different.
- Possess a vaginal pH greater than 4.5 and experience symptoms that are unabated by over-the-counter medication.

- Feel you may have contracted a sexually transmitted infection (STI) observe a yellow or bloody discharge, or discharge that smells bad, have additional symptoms such as fever, vomiting, or stomach and low back pain.
- Experience trouble peeing or need to urinate more frequently than normal

You might not need to schedule an appointment if you have experienced a yeast infection in the past and are aware of the symptoms. Yeast infections are frequently treated at home with over-the-counter drugs.

However, if you see a doctor or other healthcare professional frequently, it never hurts to get in touch with them. They might be able to help you identify the cause and recommend a course of action that works better. If you're unsure about the kind of infection you have, you should schedule an appointment as well.

If you are pregnant or suspect you may be pregnant, you should always seek medical attention from a physician or other qualified healthcare professional for any vaginal infection. If left untreated, vaginal infections can worsen and in certain cases cause issues with pregnancy and delivery.

What would happen if you got an infection?

You can't always treat a vaginal infection at home, even though some do go away with time, over-the-counter medications, and home remedies. Antibiotics or prescription antifungal drugs are necessary for treating certain infections.

If you have any of the following conditions, a medical expert can provide additional advice on locating a suitable treatment and avoiding further infections:

- Any fresh or worrisome symptoms
- Signs that do not go away or an infection that returns
- Vaginal infections, when left untreated, can be extremely uncomfortable, but they are typically not dangerous. They usually get better fast if you get the proper diagnosis and care.

Chapter 7: Giving Your Vagina a Joyful Home

Despite being owned by about 50% of us, the vagina—whatever you choose to call yours—is more mysterious and taboo than any other body part.

Though it can also be a source of shame and worry for people all over the world (45% of Westerners with vaginas never discuss their health with anyone, not even their doctor), the vagina is also what gives life itself, joy, and pleasure.

We have so much time for a new book that aims to embrace vaginas in all their glory because it is so important to be able to talk about your vagina in all its glory and without shame. This is why it is so important for you to be able to take control of your health and pleasure.

We are so excited about this Book of Vagina's mission to normalize discourse about the vagina, dispel stigmas, and celebrate what makes our intimate organs so amazing.

You'll learn from this that women's lack of confidence is not only making them hesitant to discuss their intimate areas with doctors, but it's also seriously affecting . their romantic relationships. Over two thirds of millennial vagina owners have declined oral sex due to vaginal self-consciousness, according to research. That is a great deal of enjoyment lost. Anna has compiled the following five steps to fall in love with your vagina if you're feeling self-critical. These steps are for everyone to follow.

Take a look at it!

Lack of self-esteem is the biggest barrier facing vagina owners, but given that 44% of women are unable to recognize the vagina on a medical diagram, many of us also feel self-conscious about an area we have never seen well. I advise you to get a mirror, spread your legs wide, and examine your vagina closely. Spread your labia gently and enjoy its rich colors and delicate shape. You are flawless, and this is who you are," she exclaimed.

Gazing at your vagina is not only empowering, but it's also essential for maintaining your health. It's critical to understand what is normal for your vagina and to be well-aware of your appearance, so you'll be able to detect problems quickly."

Practice loving yourself.

Let's be clear: there is no negative aspect, risk, or harm connected to masturbating, despite centuries of stigma, taboo, and shame. It feels fantastic, is healthy, and is natural.

It can significantly alter your feelings about your vagina to reframe it as something that can provide pleasure instead of concentrating on its appearance, advises Anna.

Masturbation has several health benefits, such as reducing stress, relieving period pain, and improving sleep quality. Furthermore, a ménage à moil won't only improve your health. Frequent masturbation boosts your sexual confidence and raises your chances of having an orgasm with a partner."

Make a playlist for vagina.

Lyrics about the vagina can provide a great sense of empowerment, according to Anna. Pour a drink and turn up the volume for your very own vagina-themed party, whether you're rapping along with Doja Cat, dancing to Charli XCX, or bopping to Cyndi Lauper. These are the tunes she recommends:

Discuss your vagina.

According to Anna, having a conversation about your vagina in a comfortable setting is the best way to feel good about it. "In opening up about your downstairs, you'll be taking the first step to eliminating the shame and taboo that prevents so many vagina-owners from seeking help and reassurance when they need it," she continued.

Many women, even when talking to their doctors, find it uncomfortable to talk about their vaginal health, according to studies. More than 20% of women ages 35 and under say they would not get a smear test, and more than half of them are unable to correctly label a diagram of their genitalia.

"Try confiding in someone you can trust, even if it's just by telling a joke, talking about a concern you have, or using the term "vagina" instead of "private parts." You'll be astounded at how much talking candidly about your body can boost your self-esteem ", the speaker stated.

Recognize the power of the vagina.

You can find solace in the knowledge that your vagina loves itself, even if you haven't yet learned to love it. Ladies, vaginas are self-care experts.

As Anna explains: "A complete colony of beneficial bacteria that produce lactic acid makes the vagina their home during puberty. The vagina is shielded from infections by the acidity these bacteria produce there. Your discharge has actually bleached the fabric, which is why you might notice that the gusset of your underwear gets lighter over time.

Images may include: Nature, graphics, art, and the outdoors.

"A very delicate balance exists in the vaginal ecology. In addition to discharge, this intricate system cleans the vagina automatically, requiring no effort from the vaginal owner. Every time you take a shower, swish some plain, unscented soap around the outer vulva area as a way to express gratitude to your vagina for its amazing cleaning capabilities."

It's quite remarkable, isn't it?

Do you need some last advice on how to feel confident about your genitalia? Anna ends by saying, "Your vagina. A sexy-looking, self-cleaning, miraculous device between your thighs. What a miracle. Whatever your past may have been, accept that your vagina is flawless exactly the way it is. What's the best part, then? Nobody cares what you do with your vagina—from conceiving to inducing excruciating orgasms—it's all your business."

Techniques for Having an "Extra Sweet" Vagina

Alright, allow me to state the obvious first. The reference to the next impending holiday in the title "extra sweet" is actually more of wordplay. It's Valentine's Day, as everyone is aware. I believe it is crucial to discuss this openly because I am tired of reading articles that suggest we can change the taste of our vagina to something like chocolate ice cream or a pineapple smoothie. Whoever said that to you was lying. LARGE TIME.

Nonetheless, there are undoubtedly things you can incorporate into your daily regimen to make your vulva and vagina feel fresher, less acidic, and perhaps even a little sweeter. That is what this fine day is going to be all about.

Thus, if your intention for Valentine's Day is to be your significant other's favorite person, here are a few simple tips that will elevate your relationship to a whole new level. All set?

1. **Steer Clear of These Foods**

I mean, who hasn't heard that pineapple juice tastes sweeter in the vagina? Both yes and no. Again, the truth is that no matter what we do, our hot pocket wasn't designed to taste like a fruit salad, so it won't. Having said that, it is true that our diet can affect how acidic or salty our natural lubrication is, or discharge. This is because our mucosal secretions are influenced by the food we eat.

Because of this, it's a good idea to stay away from foods that contain sulfur, such as onions and garlic (which go without saying), sugary foods (which can upset your pH balance), dairy products (which can lower immunity and alter the pH of your vagina), asparagus (which can cause a stench in urine and occasionally discharge), and red meat (which has a tendency to be high in saturated fat, which can cause bacterial infections). How long should you stay away from them? Well, starting on the Tuesday before Valentine's Day, if you're expecting a lot of oral communication, it's best to forgo these.

2. **Increase Your Water Intake**

Since water makes up between 60 and 65 percent of our bodies, we must regularly consume it. In addition to flushing out toxins and regulating body temperature, water also helps to keep us regular, boosts immunity, promotes happiness, keeps us hydrated, lessens breakouts, and increases saliva and lubrication production—all of which are critical for fellatio and cunnilingus.

This is an additional technique to keep your vagina extra fresh from the inside out because water aids in the removal of bacteria. If you decide to occasionally drink some infused water or add a few mint sprigs to your water, it can only get better.

3. **Taste Some Kefir I believe I've mentioned my sensitivity to fungi previously**. Because of this, I have experienced a higher than average number of yeast infections (not limited to my vagina; I once had a particularly nasty one under my breasts) and bouts of tinea versicolor. Nevertheless, I knew that

I needed to take a probiotic when I had a yeast infection and was prescribed an antibiotic because medications have a tendency to eradicate both good and bad bacteria; probiotics replenish the good that was eliminated (so that you don't end up with a yeast infection all over again).

You can get help with this by consuming kefir, which is essentially fermented milk with less fat. It's basically drinkable yogurt at the end of the day, before you turn up your nose. Kefir has many health benefits, including the ability to regulate blood sugar, lower cholesterol, enhance digestion, help manage weight, and maintain the health of your vagina with its antibacterial and antifungal properties. My vagina smells even better now that I've included kefir into my regular diet. I've heard from a few other customers that their partners can definitely taste the difference.

4. **Give up alcohol and coffee**.

No matter how much you enjoy wine or coffee, you should probably cut back on both of them 48 hours before Valentine's Day. Coffee's caffeine content actually depletes the vagina of the vitamins and minerals necessary for it to stay healthy. Furthermore, it has the ability to change your genitalia's odor—and not in a positive way. Spirits? Although it has the potential to boost libido, it can also cause dehydration in the body. Nobody desires a parched va-jay-jay. Thus, make an effort to cut back on alcohol in the days before V-Day. Instead, have it on the actual day.

5. **Grab a Celery Snack**

It tastes like nothing at all, celery. On that, I think we can all agree. However, keeping some in your refrigerator is a great idea so you can nibble on a few, if not more, stalks. Several times every week. On the health tip, ninety-five percent of it is water, so it can help flush out toxins and keep you hydrated. Furthermore, celery has a good supply of vitamins A, C, and K. Additionally, the calcium, iron, and magnesium in it can balance out the acids in your body. Celery also contains a good number of anti-inflammatory and antioxidant compounds. Regarding your vagina, celery can help ward off harmful bacteria because it contains vitamin C. Celery's chlorophyll will also improve the scent of your va-jay-jay.

6. **Take A Few Apple-Cherry-Cran Shots**

Nothing can replicate the taste of your vagina. And there's nothing at all wrong with that. Nevertheless, some fruits have nutrients that can enhance the pleasure and attractiveness of our vagina. Strong antioxidants found in cranberries will maintain the equilibrium of your pH levels. In addition to their anti-inflammatory properties, bing cherries also contain antioxidants. Apples are great because they increase lubrication and blood flow to the vaginal region because of the phytoestrogen phloridzin and its antioxidants. Imagine the power of this combination (use 100% juice; avoid the extra-sugary variety as it will hinder rather than help your health).

7. Take a Look at Some Frozen Grapes

Playing with temperature—that is, going from warm to cold—is incredibly stimulating when it comes to sexual stimulation. As an added bonus, how about adding some frozen grapes to the mixture? Grapes are 82 percent water and have thin skin, so your partner can tease you all over your vaginal area with them without worrying that they will irritate you days later.

You will feel amazing with a frozen grape on your clitoral hood, I promise. The grape that you are sharing will then taste amazing to you both.

8. Remember to Use Coconut and Cinnamon Oils

You couldn't convince me not to have a concoction of coconut oil and cinnamon oil on a bed stand back when I was first getting it in. Because it can safely dilute the potency of cinnamon oil and has properties to keep your vagina drama-free, coconut oil is awesome. Because it has a warming effect and tastes sweet and cinnamon, cinnamon oil is fantastic. To answer the doubters, it doesn't burn. Just remember that "less is more" when making decisions. In any case, this is a pretty unrivaled combination if you're looking for a gift that never stops.

9. **Get Some Edible Lubricant**

There are many flavored lubricants on the market that are safe to use for oral sex or anything else sex-related, if you're not ready to basically DIY your delicious lubricant. Let's Talk Sex examined 12 different brands to help you select the one that best fits your needs and preferences. Here is where you can view them all.

10. **Incorporate Rosewater into Your Bath Soap**

Rosewater can improve the flavor of things, did you know that? For this reason, it occasionally appears as an ingredient in various sauces and desserts. Rosewater has a lot of health benefits as well, including the ability to treat infections, soothe skin, and elevate mood. It's no wonder I included it in this list of methods for making your vagina smell better.

You can gently clean your vagina by adding some rosewater to your bath water. Then, your vagina will smell inviting and feminine if you dab a little of it on your outer labia before getting into something sexy. That sounds like the ideal formula for a pretty sweet 'n sexy Valentine's Day evening. Have fun. You two together.

Chapter 8: Vaginal Nutrition

Enhancing your diet with specific foods and nutrients could help your vaginal health. Find out which foods to try and which ones to avoid.

Taking good care of your nutrition is crucial to maintaining your general health. Food has an effect on the health of certain body parts, such as the vagina. Certain foods have been linked to maintaining the health of the vagina, according to research. Certain foods, for example, can help keep the vagina lubricated, while others can help prevent infection.

Top Foods for Healthy Vagina

While the best overall nutritional strategy is typically a balanced diet high in whole foods, there are some foods or nutrients that may be especially beneficial for vaginal health.

Rich in Probiotic Foods

Probiotics are live bacteria that have been shown to have a variety of health benefits, including improved immune system function and assistance with digestion. It has also been demonstrated that probiotics enhance vaginal health.

Numerous microorganisms, including beneficial bacteria like the probiotic Lactobacillus, can be found in the vagina. Sexually transmitted infections (STIs), yeast infections, and bacterial vaginosis (BV) are among the microorganisms that lactobacillus guards against. Fermented foods such as the following contain Lactobacillus-containing probiotics:

- Live cultures in yogurt
- Pickles
- Pickles with Kimchi
- Miso, or paste made from soy.
- Temper—a soy-based product
- Kombucha

You can also take these probiotics as supplements to help your vagina.

According to research, consuming probiotic supplements containing Lactobacillus can raise the bacteria's concentration in the vagina. One week after starting the supplement, the effects have been demonstrated to start. The amount of dangerous bacteria in the vagina can also be decreased by taking a probiotic supplement that contains Lactobacillus strains.

In addition to producing probiotics, antimicrobials are substances that either kill or inhibit the growth of other bacteria while also enhancing immunity in order to keep the proper balance of "good" and "harmful" bacteria in the vagina.

There has been conflicting research on the effects of probiotic supplements on vaginal health; some studies have found little to no additional benefit.

Consult a healthcare provider for advice on which probiotic-rich foods to eat or which supplements to take, as well as the recommended dosage, for vaginal health. There are no set guidelines regarding probiotic foods or supplements.

Low-GI Foods

Two-thirds of women who are of reproductive age are affected by BV, the most common gynecological disorder. A bacterial imbalance in the vagina can lead to a bacterial infection known as BV.

Vaginal odor, discharge, itching, and burning are possible signs of BV. Redness and swelling are not always present with these symptoms. BV may make STIs more likely.

Consuming low-GI foods may aid in the prevention of BV.

The glycemic index is a scale that quantifies the rate at which foods high in carbohydrates cause glucose, or sugars, to enter the bloodstream and raise blood sugar levels. Foods with a low glycemic index release glucose gradually, which can aid in regulating blood sugar levels.

Foods with a low glycemic index include, for example:

- Complete grains such as barley, quinoa, and oatmeal

Among the non-starchy vegetables are carrots.

- Fruits such as grapefruit, oranges, and apples
- Most legumes, beans, and nuts
- Yogurt Made with Milk

Foods with a high glycemic index swiftly release glucose, elevating blood sugar levels. This could raise the chance of BV.

It's unclear exactly how BV and glucose levels relate to one another. According to one theory, high blood sugar levels can weaken the immune system, promote inflammation, and promote the growth of bacteria in the vaginal fluids.

High-Fibre Meals

Consuming foods high in fiber may encourage the growth of Lactobacillus, a bacterium that colonizes the vagina and controls harmful bacteria. Increased fiber consumption may also aid in the prevention of BV.

High-fiber foods include:

- Complete grains such as barley, quinoa, and oatmeal
- Most legumes, nuts, seeds, and beans

- Boiled artichokes
- Sweet potatoes that have been cooked

Berries along with other types of fruits

One easy way to increase your intake of dietary fiber is to eat more whole grains. Here are some ideas for replacing whole grains with refined ones:

- Use only whole grain bread in place of white bread.
- Use only whole grain pasta in place of regular pasta.
- Pick oatmeal instead of baked goods or muffins for breakfast.
- Instead of using white rice, use quinoa or brown rice.
- Items Rich in Vitamin D
- Vitamin D is another important nutrient that might assist with a few aspects of vaginal health.

Vitamin D is present in:

- Salmon that has been cooked
- Trout
- Eggs with Sardines
- Milks supplemented with D
- Cheese cheddar

Getting enough vitamin D every day from food alone can be difficult. To reach the daily recommended levels, a lot of people might take supplements.

A review published in 2022 suggests that vitamin D may help women going through menopause by balancing the pH levels in the vagina, reducing dryness in the vagina, and enhancing the diversity and growth of cells in the vaginal lining. All of these things can contribute to the vagina's general health being better. More research is necessary, though, as there hasn't been much of it.

Those with low blood levels of vitamin D may benefit from taking an extra dosage of the vitamin each day to help treat BV. This is due to the fact that vitamin D has the potential to strengthen the immune system, which may support general vaginal health.

Apples

According to some research, apples may promote normal sexual function. According to one study, women who ate one or more apples a day reported better vaginal lubrication and higher levels of sexual satisfaction than those who ate fewer than one.

To improve the health of your vagina: Increase your intake of apples.

Chopped apples can be added to garden salads, yogurt, oatmeal, and smoothies.

Slices of apple are dipped in nut butter.

Add thinly sliced apples to stir fries and slaws.

For a dessert with less sugar, bake apples.

Foods to Avoid

Limiting highly processed foods is one way to maintain vaginal health.

According to one study, eating foods high in sugar, solid fats, red meat, fried potatoes, refined grains, and organ meats on a regular basis is significantly linked to an increased risk of BV.

Foods with a high glycemic index have been found to raise the risk of BV.

Glycemic index-high foods include:

- White bread and bagels
- Processed grains found in snack foods, instant oatmeal, and sugary cereals
- White rice
- Sugar and Honey

To steer clear of highly processed foods, opt for healthy meals like stir-fries, salads, and soups that include vegetables, lean protein, and whole grains. As a snack, enjoy fresh fruit and nuts or veggies with hummus.

A Brief Recap

The condition of your vagina can be influenced by specific foods or nutrients. High-fiber foods may help prevent BV, foods high in probiotics may help control the microorganisms in your vagina, and apples may help keep your vagina lubricated. Your vaginal health may also be impacted by the general quality of your diet. For instance, a diet heavy in processed foods may increase the risk of BV.

It's unlikely that food will be enough to treat or prevent infections or other ailments. Speak with a healthcare professional about any concerns you have regarding your vaginal health, and find out if food has any place in any proposed treatment plan.

Chapter 9: Improving Intimacy and Sexual Satisfaction

How can I increase the intimacy and sexual gratification I get from a relationship?

Enhance intimacy and sexual satisfaction by:

1. Being transparent in discussing goals and limits.

2. Giving emotional support and quality time top priority.

3. Experimenting with new hobbies and ideas as a group.

4. Acquiring knowledge of one another's physical attributes.

5. Going slow and putting enjoyment rather than performance first.

How can I increase the intimacy and sexual gratification I get from a relationship?

Boost intimacy and sexual satisfaction by:

Discussing boundaries and desires in an honest manner.

Putting quality time and emotional connection first.

Together, we explore new interests and fantasies.

Gaining knowledge of and respect for one another's bodies.

Slowing down and putting enjoyment above performance.

Developing a solid and healthy connection with your partner can be greatly aided by increasing sexual satisfaction and intimacy in a partnership.

The following advice could be helpful:

1. **Communication**: In order to have a fulfilling sexual relationship, open and honest communication is essential. Discuss your likes, dislikes, and any worries you may have with your partner. Be willing to hear what your partner needs to say.

2. **Experimentation**: Trying new things in the bedroom can help keep things interesting and novel. Examine each other's bodies and experiment with various poses and methods.

3. **Foreplay**: Engaging in foreplay can improve sex pleasure and help both partners get into the right frame of mind.

4. **Put the pleasure first**: Explore each other's bodies and enjoy the experience rather than concentrating only on orgasm.

5. **Look after yourself**: Having a positive self-image can increase your level of sexual satisfaction and confidence. Make sure you're physically, mentally, and emotionally healthy.

Ways to enhance your sexual life

Your general state of mental, physical, and emotional well-being is closely linked to your sexual well-being. Regardless of the problems you're having, there are plenty of things you can do to improve your sexual life and have more satisfying relationships.

Having a fulfilling sexual life

Sexual. A wide range of emotions can be evoked by the word. The emotions evoked by sexual experiences range widely, from longing, anxiety, and disappointment to love, excitement, and tenderness. Furthermore, during the course of a decades-long sexual life, many people will experience all of these feelings in addition to many others.

However, what exactly is sex?

Sex is essentially just another hormone-driven biological process meant to ensure the survival of the species. That limited perspective, of course, undervalues the complexity of the sexual response in humans. Your experiences and expectations, along with the biochemical factors at play, contribute to the formation of your sexual identity. A fulfilling sexual life is largely dependent on your perception of yourself as a sexual being, your ideas about what makes a satisfying sexual connection and your relationship with your partner.

Speaking with your spouse

Even in ideal situations, many couples find it difficult to have a sexual conversation. Feelings of hurt, guilt, shame, and resentment can completely stop a conversation when sexual problems arise. Starting a conversation is the first step to a better sex life as well as a stronger emotional connection because effective communication is the foundation of a healthy relationship. Here are some pointers for dealing with this delicate matter.

Choose the ideal moment to speak. Sexual conversations can be divided into two categories: those that take place in the bedroom and those that take place outside of it. While it's acceptable to share intimate information with your partner during a passionate moment, it's preferable to postpone discussing more serious matters, like mismatched sexual desires or orgasm difficulties, until you're in a more neutral environment.

Refrain from criticizing. Instead of concentrating on the drawbacks, couch suggestions in positive terms, like "I really love it when you touch my hair lightly that way." Instead of using a sexual issue as an opportunity to place blame, approach it as a problem that needs to be solved jointly.

Tell your spouse about the changes you've noticed in your body. Discuss these issues with your partner if hot flashes are preventing you from sleeping at night or if menopause has left your vagina dry. Rather than taking these physical changes as a sign of disinterest, it would be much better if he knew what was actually going on. Similarly, if you're a man and you can't get an erection at the mere mention of having sex, teach your partner how to arouse you instead of allowing her to think she's not attractive enough.

Be truthful. By pretending to have an orgasm, you may believe that you are safeguarding your partner's feelings, but in actuality, you are taking a risk. Even though discussing any sexual issue can be difficult, things get much harder when the problem is hidden under years of deceit, hurt, and bitterness.

Never confuse love with having sex.

Establish a tender and loving environment by touching and kissing frequently. Your inability to have sex is not your partner's or your own fault. Instead, concentrate on preserving your relationship's emotional and physical closeness. What will happen when one partner passes away is a potentially delicate topic worth discussing for older couples. In relationships where there is a healthy sexual life, the survivor will probably want to look for a new partner. While you are both still alive, expressing your openness to that possibility will probably ease guilt and ease the process for the surviving partner afterwards.

Applying self-help techniques

Today, treating sexual problems is simpler than in the past. Expert sex therapists and cutting-edge drugs are available if you need them. However, you might be able to fix minor sexual problems by changing the way you make love. Here are a few ideas for at-home experiments.

Learn for yourself. For any kind of sexual problem, there are a plethora of excellent self-help resources available. Look through the Internet or your neighborhood bookshop, select a few resources that speak to you, and use them to educate yourself and your partner on the issue. If having a direct conversation is too tough, you and your partner can highlight and show each other the passages you find particularly interesting.

Take your time. Your sexual arousal decreases with age. You can increase your chances of success with your partner by finding a peaceful, cozy, and distraction-free place to have sex. Recognize that it will take longer for you to become aroused and experience an orgasm due to the physical changes in your body. If you think about it, having more sex isn't always a bad thing.

Incorporating these physical requirements into your routine can lead to new and exciting sexual experiences.

Apply lubricant. Using lubricating liquids and gels, it is frequently possible to easily treat the dry vagina that appears during the perimenopause. Use them freely to steer clear of uncomfortable sexual encounters, which can lead to a waning libido and escalating conflict in relationships. Talk with your doctor about other options if lubricants are no longer effective.

Continue to show physical affection. Keeping up an emotional and physical bond requires kissing and cuddling, even when you're worn out, stressed, or angry about the issue.

Practice making contact. Sex therapists can assist you in reestablishing physical intimacy without putting you under pressure by using sensate focus techniques. These exercises have many variations found in self-help books and instructional videos. Asking your partner to touch you in a way that suits him or her might also be a good idea. This will help you determine how much pressure—from light to heavy—you should apply.

Try assuming various positions. Having a repertoire of various sexual positions not only makes making love more interesting, but it can also be useful in resolving conflict. For instance, the G-spot's heightened stimulation that happens when a man helps the woman experience an orgasm by approaching his partner from behind.

Jot down your dreams. You can use this exercise to investigate activities that you and your partner might find interesting. Try recalling an incident or a movie that made you feel agitated, then tell your partner about it. Those with low desire will particularly benefit from this.

Perform Kegel exercises. Exercise of the pelvic floor muscles can enhance sexual fitness in both sexes. Tighten the same muscle that you would use to stop pee in midstream in order to perform these exercises. After two or three seconds of holding the contraction, release it. Ten times over, repeat. Aim for five sets each day. You can perform these exercises while standing in a checkout line, driving, or sitting at your desk. Women who want to increase muscle resistance at home can use vaginal weights. For information on where to obtain and how to use these, consult your physician or a sex therapist.

Make an effort to unwind. Play a game or go out to a nice dinner as a relaxing activity to do before having sex. Alternatively, attempt methods of relaxation like yoga or deep breathing exercises.

Make use of a vibrator. With the use of this tool, a woman can better understand her own sexual response and communicate her preferences to her partner.

Remain persistent. Don't give up if it seems like nothing you try will work. Your physician is frequently in a position to identify the root cause of your sexual issue as well as potential therapies. Additionally, he or she can connect you with a sex therapist who can assist you in exploring problems that might be preventing you from having fulfilling relationships.

The G-mark

The G-spot, also known as the Grafenberg spot after the gynecologist who first discovered it, is a lump of extremely sensitive sponge-like tissue that is situated inside the vaginal roof, directly inside the opening. Strong orgasms can be experienced when the G-spot is properly stimulated. Because of its location's difficulty and the fact that manual stimulation works best, most women do not regularly activate the G-spot during vaginal intercourse. Although this has caused some doubters to question its existence, studies have shown that this site does contain a distinct type of tissue.

To find your G-spot, you need to be sexually aroused. To locate it, try beckoningly rubbing your finger along the roof of your vagina while sitting or squatting, or have your partner massage the vagina's upper surface until you feel a particularly sensitive spot. While some women have a tendency to be more sensitive and have no trouble finding the right place, others struggle.

You shouldn't be concerned if you have trouble finding it. Many women believe that the easiest way to stimulate the G-spot during sex is for a man to approach from behind. Playing with the G-spot can help couples who are having erection issues enhance their romantic moments.

A woman may experience an extremely strong orgasm if she gets both manual and oral stimulation of the G-spot.

Preserving Health

Your general state of mental, physical, and emotional well-being is closely linked to your sexual well-being. Thus, you can shape up your sex life with the same healthy habits that help you maintain your physical appearance.

Exercise is essential. The most important healthy habit that can enhance your sexual functioning is physical activity. Aerobic exercise is essential because it strengthens your heart and blood vessels, which is necessary for proper blood flow, which is a major factor in physical arousal. In addition, exercise has a plethora of other health advantages, such as preventing heart disease, osteoporosis, and some types of cancer, elevating your mood, and promoting sounder sleep. Remember to incorporate strength training as well.

Avoid smoking. Peripheral vascular disease, which impacts blood flow to the penis, clitoris, and vaginal tissues, is exacerbated by smoking. Moreover, women who smoke typically experience menopause two years earlier than their non-smoking peers. Try nicotine gum or patches, or talk to your doctor about the medications varenicline (Chantix) and bupropion (Zyban) if you need assistance stopping.

Drink alcohol sparingly. While a single drink may help some erectile dysfunction sufferers unwind, abusing alcohol can exacerbate the condition. Alcohol dulls the central nervous system, which can prevent sexual reflexes. Men who drink heavily and for an extended period of time may produce more estrogen because of liver damage. Alcohol can exacerbate menopausal symptoms in women by causing hot flashes and sleep disturbances.

Consume healthfully. Overindulgence in fat-containing foods results in obesity and elevated blood cholesterol, two major risk factors for cardiovascular disease. Overweight can also encourage a negative body image and apathy. One additional benefit of losing those extra pounds is frequently an increase in libido.

Make use of it or discard it. The vaginal walls lose some of their elasticity when estrogen levels drop during menopause. Through sexual activity, you can halt or even reverse this process. If having sex isn't an option, masturbation works just as well. For women, though, it works best if you use a vibrator or dildo, which is a penis-like device, to help stretch the vagina. Men who go extended periods without having an erection may lose some of the blood that is rich in oxygen that the penis needs to function properly during sexual activity. This causes muscle cells to produce tissue that resembles scar tissue, which prevents the penis from expanding in response to an increase in blood flow.

Reviving the fun in sexual relations

After a while, sex can become boring, even in the best of relationships. You just need to use a little creativity to reignite the flame.

Take risks and be bold. Perhaps now is the perfect time to try having sex in a private area of the woods or on the floor of your living room. Or look into sensual movies and books. You might feel flirtatious just from the sense of misbehavior you get when you rent an X-rated film.

Exhibit sensuality. Make love in a setting that satisfies all five of your senses. Feel the silk against your skin, the rhythm of a jazz song, the aroma of flowers filling the space, the gentle glow of a candle, and the flavor of ripe, juicy fruit. Make use of your increased awareness of sensuality when you make love to your partner.

Play around. Put notes of affection in your partner's pocket for them to discover at a later time. Have a bubble bath together; the sensation of warmth and coziness you experience after stepping out of the tub can be a wonderful prelude to sex. Snicker. Laugh.

Use your imagination. Increase the variety of your sexual scripts and your repertory. If you usually make love on Saturday night, for instance, consider choosing Sunday morning. Try out different roles and pursuits. If you have never tried sex toys and sexy lingerie, give them a try.

Show some romance. Sing poetry aloud to one another on a hillside beneath a tree. Give each other flowers as a surprise when there's no special occasion. Schedule a day where you just talk, cuddle, and lie in bed. The most valuable resource at your disposal is your perspective on sexuality. If you have a positive attitude and solid information, you should be able to continue having healthy relationships for a long time.

Chapter 10: The benefits of physical intimacy and the mind-body connection

Many health benefits of sex exist. Studies on the relationship between the mind and body reveal that our emotions can affect our physical health and vice versa. Intimate sexual relationships can elicit positive emotions that may also contribute to our physical well-being.

Research has demonstrated that regular sex has advantages beyond the benefits of intimacy in a loving relationship. These advantages include:

- Amelioration of mood
- Alleviation of depression
- Reduction of stress
- A greater sense of wellbeing and self-worth
- Elevations in the hormone oxytocin, which is connected to happier moods and better sleep
- Elevated endorphin levels, which lessen overall pain perception

Intimacy and symptoms of IBD

Physical signs and symptoms

The nausea, diarrhea, cramps in the abdomen, and vomiting that are frequently experienced by those who have Crohn's or colitis are well-known to most people. Long-term companions will also be acquainted with them. Fistulas, or "tunnels" of infection that can form in the intestine and tunnel to the skin or a nearby organ, are another physical sign of Crohn's disease or colitis. Due to tearing, a fistula in the anal or vaginal regions may hurt during intercourse.

Your doctor, your partner, and you may be able to jointly manage it in the short- and/or long-term, depending on your physical symptoms.

When you meet with your healthcare provider, be honest and open with them. Take the time to explain in detail how the symptoms affect intimate acts. Your supplier might have some ideas.

Symptoms of the mind and body

Crohn's disease and colitis physical symptoms can affect your emotional state, resulting in weariness, apathy, and possibly even depression. Depressive symptoms can lessen one's sense of desirability or worth.

The good news is that you can treat some of these problems on your own or in conjunction with your healthcare team.

Strategies for Adjusting

Evaluate your immediate capabilities and have a conversation with them. Although you might think that your date or partner will only accept sexual activity, they might be flexible and willing to try anything at that point. Invite him or her to share their thoughts and desires with you as well as to have an honest and open discussion about sexual activities.

Don't completely give up on intimacy either; body massages, hugs, kisses, and other physical affections can all improve your physical well-being. Beyond engaging in sexual activity, you two can do a lot together (penetrative sex).

Being open to trying out and participating in different kinds of physical intimacy may boost your desire and boost your confidence, which will reduce your reluctance to get close.

Be mindful of your self-talk regarding your diagnosis: do you treat your body with kindness or with criticism? Are you asking more of yourself than your body can handle? Celebrate what your body can accomplish despite having Crohn's or colitis, just like you would with a close friend. Positive body image makes you feel good about your physical appearance, which opens up doors to intimacy.

The vagina is not just a sex organ; rather, it is a potent mediator of female confidence, creativity, and the sense of connections between things.

THIS PLEASURE PRINCIPLE:
THE BRAIN AND VAGINAL CONNECTION

In my capacity as a women's wellness consultant and sacred sex educator, I often consider how women view themselves as sexual beings. Usually, I'm interested in how we view our bodies and sex. Based on my interactions with women at retreats and workshops, I have observed that women typically don't know a lot about our bodies and how they function. Although we are generally aware of the anatomy of our sex, there is still much more for us to learn.

Having sex is vital to a healthy lifestyle. Science has shown that having sex is not only beneficial for the endocrine system (hormone network) but also for your general feelings of joy, peace, creativity, and happiness. The "pleasure cocktail" of hormones released during good sex is dopamine, opioids, and oxytocin. You may be asexual, the victim of uneventful sex, or have experienced sexual trauma if, as you read this, you're reflecting on how your past sexual experiences have left you feeling less than joyful and creative. Since my intention is never to minimize any of our experiences, but rather to raise awareness so that we can unlock the goodness that is stored in our bodies, I want to validate your feelings and your experiences.

The human body is designed to be a vehicle for pleasure. Consider the fact that the clitoris serves only one purpose, which is pleasure.

It seems that researchers have been doing some pretty amazing work, finding compelling evidence to back up the theories of old philosophy, like Hindu Tantra and Kemetic. The vagina and brain are linked; in fact, author and journalist Naomi Wolf refers to them as a "single system." In her book Vagina: A New Biography, she makes this claim.

When properly understood, female sexual pleasure transcends both sexuality and pleasure. Additionally, it functions as a medium for feminine self-awareness and optimism, feminine bravery and inventiveness, feminine initiative and focus, feminine transcendence and bliss, and feminine sensibility that strongly suggests freedom. Realizing that the vagina is not only coextensive with the female brain but also fundamentally a component of the female soul is necessary to comprehend the vagina properly.

This is a really significant claim. A woman is more likely to feel and be better after having healthy sex and feeling secure and protected. Feeling safe is crucial for women in this situation. To experience what mystics refer to as cosmic bliss, we need to feel secure and connected in order to enter an altered state of consciousness. Sex is supposed to be a wonderful, healing, creative, and ecstasy-filled experience.

This means that we need to know ourselves and always be willing to learn more. To ensure the most enjoyable experiences, we must be dedicated to working only with people who can facilitate the development of the best possible connections.

It is both a gift and a natural right to be happy. Obtain some for yourself!

www.ingramcontent.com/pod-product-compliance
Lightning Source LLC
Chambersburg PA
CBHW070851260726
48661CB00004B/1345